Rockin' Robin's Handbook to a Healthier Life

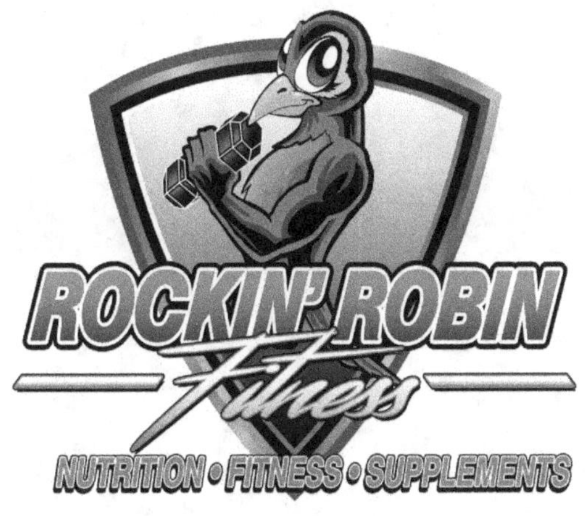

Robin Lacagnina

Certified Personal Trainer

Disclaimer
Any similarities to existing recipes are purely coincidental

To all of you who are willing to put in a little extra time and effort to live a healthier life

To my husband and my children Matthew, Brian, Nicole & Anthony who bring me the greatest joy, with love

Acknowledgements

I'd like to thank my husband Peter for making this all possible. I'd like to thank him for his endless support of Rockin' Robin Fitness and his endless support of me.

I'd like to thank my four amazing children for your support and encouragement. On any given day, there is a good chance that one of you (if not all of you) are wearing a Rockin' Robin tee shirt, sweatshirt, or shorts.

I'd like to thank all the special people in my life that helped and inspired me along the way, you know who you are.

Thanks to my clients, past, present, and future, for allowing me to do what I love to do with people I love to be with. How lucky am I?

Thanks to all my friends and family who have ever had to eat a meal with me. Thanks for making special foods for me and thanks for dealing with my substitutions when we go out.

In the world of health and fitness, things are always changing. The information that I will share with you in this book is based on the information that was available to me at the time of writing.

It is my desire that you use the information in this book as a foundation and that you continue to grow and learn as more information becomes available. When it comes to your health, knowledge is power.

People in earlier generations were not as fortunate as we are to have all of this information available. We have the information now, and we need only incorporate it into our lives and continue to stay educated on the latest research in order to make the most out of the quality of our lives.

Before starting an exercise program, it is recommended that you consult with your physician.

Table of Contents

Chapter 1

Rockin' Robin Fitness

My Story

Rockin' Robin Fitness

My initial motivation for becoming a certified personal trainer was to help my clients achieve a better-looking body. However, through my education at International Fitness Professionals Association (IFPA), I have discovered that improving your waistline is actually just a bonus. Now, my primary goal as a certified personal trainer is to enhance the quality of life for my clients as they age.

Aging is inevitable, but exercise can be very helpful! For example, exercise can help reduce the risk of osteoporosis, a disease that makes bones become fragile and more likely to break. Also as we age, we lose approximately five pounds of muscle mass every ten years. Each pound of muscle requires about thirty-five to fifty additional calories daily in order to maintain that muscle. Each pound of fat burns only two to three calories a day. It may not seem like a lot, but over time it adds up.

We often hear people complain about aches and pains as they age. Many of the aches and pains felt later on in life are actually caused by muscle atrophy, or decrease in muscle mass. Exercise, with its ability to build and maintain muscle, is essential to improving the quality of your life. It reduces the risk of adult onset diabetes, colon cancer, and heart disease. In addition, exercise may reduce blood pressure and cholesterol, while increasing muscle mass and boosting metabolic function.

There are three components to improving the quality of your life: a healthy diet, cardiovascular training, and strength training. I challenge you to take control of your future today. Start with a brisk walk and start planning a fitness routine that works for your lifestyle.

My Story

Up until I was in my late thirties, I was a big junk-food eater. I would think nothing of having cookies for breakfast. I could go days without a vegetable. But as I learned more and more about fitness, I realized that if I wanted to continue to live a healthy life, a cookie for breakfast was no longer an option. I needed to make serious changes.

I made a new life resolution to change my eating habits. It was April when I came to this conclusion, so I wasn't waiting for January to make a New Year's resolution. If you want to make life changes badly enough, you can start today.

Improving my eating habits was *not* easy. The first few days were challenging, but I managed to get through them. Then the weekend came and I was at a party. Although I was tempted to eat the chips and other snacks, I picked at a vegetable platter instead. The real problem came when dessert was served. At the hostess's request, I had brought Dunkin' Donuts (Boston Cream, my favorite) and there was a delicious-looking cake on the table. Before I made my resolution I would probably have had a piece of each. And being at a party, I felt I was entitled to have one, but I would no longer have both. The question was, which one would I have? So I thought long and hard because I did not want to regret that very serious decision—Boston Cream donut or chocolate cake? I kept going back and forth between the two desserts. I spent so much time agonizing over this decision that the next thing I knew, everyone was done with dessert. So, I decided I was too, and I passed on dessert.

That was a turning point for me. I had no dessert at a party. I could hardly believe that I was actually able to do that. Before then, the longest I had ever gone without dessert was about two and a half weeks, but NEVER at a party. I knew that if I could pass on dessert at a party and feel great about it, I could really make this change in my life. I've been to many parties since then and have passed on many desserts (not all). When I do have a dessert, it is always just one dessert and it is a small portion.

Instead of bringing donuts to a party, now I bring a fruit salad or I bake my own healthy desserts, which is time-consuming, but well worth it. I changed some of the ingredients in my banana bread to make it healthier. I have a pumpkin muffin recipe as well as a zucchini and carrot muffin recipe. Sometimes I make extra and freeze them for future cravings. That is my new dessert and I really do enjoy it. See chapter eight for some of my healthy recipes.

My two favorite things have always been amazing deserts and great clothing. I am now at the age where I can no longer have both. I can either feel great in my clothing all day or I can enjoy a great snack that only lasts a few minutes. So, I usually opt to feel better in my clothing, and when I don't, I usually regret it.

Go ahead and make the choice to feel good all day instead of just for a few minutes. Before you know it you'll feel great all week, and then all month. Clothing may not be the thing that motivates you, but whatever your motivation may be, use it to help you achieve this very rewarding goal.

What I Believe

Health is a gift. Don't take it for granted.

Although there are times when ignorance is bliss, ignorance is not bliss when it comes to your health.

You can retrain your taste buds. Just be patient, it will take some time; just don't give up.

No food tastes so good that it's worth gambling your health for.

The way you treat your body today will have a large impact on how your body treats you tomorrow.

Nothing is as fun when you're sick. What are you doing to avoid an illness?

When it comes to weight loss, slow and steady wins the race.

Healthy food does taste good!

Exercise makes you feel proud and confident.

Exercise really can be fun.

It's never too late to start living a healthier life.

Strong mind (willpower) + strong muscles (exercise) = a great body.

The fountain of youth is accessible to all of us.

Weight loss is an added bonus to exercise and eating right. The greatest gift is improved health and fitness.

You don't have to be an athlete to be fit.

Our food is our fuel. What kind of fuel are you putting in your body?

If you're going to exercise, make it count. Don't just go through the motions!

I believe that you are worth the time and effort to live a healthier, happier life. Do you?

Everything is not okay in moderation! You wouldn't eat arsenic in moderation and you shouldn't be consuming certain toxins that ARE in our foods, even if only in moderation.

Chapter 2

Diet, Exercise &

The Quality of Your Life

Jack LaLanne

If you think that diet and exercise aren't essential for a superior quality of life, take a look at Jack LaLanne. Jack will celebrate his 96th birthday this year and he is as active as ever.

Jack wasn't always the fitness guru we all know today. As a child he was addicted to sugar. The sugar addiction caused him to be extremely violent. At one point he was so weak that his doctor advised him to stay home from school so he could "rest and regain his strength."

When Jack was about fifteen years old, a nutritionist told him that he was a human garbage can. That is when Jack went on the strict diet that he follows today. His diet consists primarily of fruits, vegetables, and fish. Jack also started an exercise routine. His philosophy is, "You've got to work at living because dying is easy." Jack asks, "Would you get your dog up in the morning and give him a cigarette, a cup of coffee and a doughnut?" The American Dietetic Association states that breakfast is the most important meal of the day. So I ask, What did you have for breakfast this morning?

Jack LaLanne hosted the first televised exercise show, starting in 1951. At seventy, Jack pulled seventy boats across the Long Beach, California, harbor with seventy people in each of them—while swimming with handcuffs. In his nineties, Jack is still working out on a regular basis. Jack took control of his life and look at the benefits he is still enjoying.

Unfortunately, the rest of Jack LaLanne's generation was not as informed about the importance of diet and exercise to quality of life as Jack was in the 1930s; but we are today. So put down the sugar cookies and grab an apple, after all, an apple a day *can* keep than the doctor away. Replace your sugary snacks with some fresh fruits and vegetables. And of course, start a fitness program; Jack didn't get his muscular physique on diet alone.

Here are some more of Jack LaLanne's personal quotes that I think are great!

*I can't die. It would ruin my image.

*If man made it, don't eat it.

*Whereas Billy Graham is all about the hereafter, I'm all about the here and now.

*Exercise is king and diet is queen; put them together and you've got an empire.

*You eat every day, you sleep every day, and your body was made to exercise every day.

There is no time like the present to start eating right and exercising. Like Jack says, you have to work at living because dying is easy! You'll be glad you did if you get the opportunity to celebrate your 96th birthday. It's a quality of life issue. Strive to make your quality of life as good as Jack's!

The Fitness Equation

Being fit is not as simple as one plus one; it's more like one plus one plus one. The reason is that there are three parts to the fitness equation. To achieve optimal health benefits, you have to incorporate all three parts into your lifestyle.

The 1st part of the equation is aerobic exercise. Aerobic exercise increases your body's demand for oxygen, thereby strengthening your heart and lungs and improving blood flow. It may reduce your risk of developing hypertension (high blood pressure), and may lower hypertension if it is already elevated. Aerobics may reduce your risk of developing cancers. Aerobic activity also stimulates and boosts your immune system, making you less susceptible to viruses. Aerobic activity can also reduce your risk of stroke, increase "good" cholesterol and decrease "bad" cholesterol. The bonus is that you will also burn fat.

The 2nd part of the equation is strength training. Strength training is important for both men and women. It improves glucose metabolism, which will decrease your risk of developing adult onset diabetes (Type 2 diabetes). It may decrease your risk of colon cancer and reduce resting blood pressure. Weight training has been shown to ease the pain of osteoarthritis and rheumatoid arthritis. Studies show that people with lower back pain had less pain after ten weeks of strength training for the back. The strength training bonus is that adding three pounds of muscle mass may increase your resting metabolism by 7 percent, which leads to weight loss. Your appetite will also increase slightly, which is why the third part of this equation is so very important.

The 3rd part of the equation is diet. A low-fat high-fiber diet is extremely important for good health. You really are what you eat! Try to avoid processed foods as much as possible, including fast food, foods that contain high fructose corn syrup, and foods made with partially hydrogenated oils. Substitute whole grain bread for white breads. Add leafy greens to your diet, they contain high amounts of folate which may reduce one's risk of getting colorectal, ovarian, and breast cancers. In just three months of changing my eating habits, my risk of coronary heart disease went from 3.7 to 3.0. In addition to the health benefits, the bonus is that you will lose fat. Other than a little fat, what do you have to lose?

Are You in Search of the Fountain of Youth?

People have been in search of the fountain of youth since 1513, when the explorer Ponce de Leon organized an expedition to find the fountain of youth. He traveled from Spain to Florida in search of this miraculous fountain. He was unsuccessful. In 1521 he set sail again in search of the fountain of youth.

Ponce de Leon never did find the fountain of youth. Neither did anyone else—or did we? All this time the power to live a more youthful life may have been within our grasp all along. I don't dismiss the role of genetics, but we do have some control over how old we feel, how old we look, and how old we act.

Following you will see some of the effects that aging has on our bodies versus the benefits that exercise has on our bodies. Take a look and then decide if there really is a fountain of youth—one that is accessible to all of us.

Effects of Aging vs. Benefits of Exercise

Effects of Aging	Benefits of Exercise
Increases Blood Pressure	Decreases Blood pressure
Increased risk of Osteoporosis	Decreased risk of osteoporosis
Decreases Muscle Mass	Increases Muscle Mass
Decreases Mental Ability	Increases Mental Ability
Decreases Sex Drive	Increases Sex Drive
Increases Cholesterol Levels	Decreases Cholesterol Levels
Decreases Metabolism	Increases Metabolism
Decreases Joint Strength	Increases Joint Strength
Decreases Flexibility	Increases Flexibly
Decreases Balance	Increases Balance
Decreases Endurance	Increases Endurance

Here are a few changes that have been reported to add years to your life, according to IFPA:

Exercise — Exercise controls the release of stress hormones, which can add an additional twenty years to your life by rejuvenating your heart, lungs, liver, and boosting your immune system.

Eat grapes — By eating grapes, which are full of flavonoids, an antioxidant found in plants, you can lower your risk of cancer, stroke, heart disease, and brain illnesses. The flavonoids in grapes slow down the aging of the arteries.

Eat nuts too — By eating just a small handful of nuts daily, you may decrease the risk of heart disease by as much as 24 percent. Nuts contain healthy fats, which can lower your cholesterol and prevent plaque buildup in arteries.

Eat tomato sauce — Tomatoes are filled with lycopene which are another antioxidant. Cooked tomatoes have seven times more lycopene than raw tomatoes. Lycopene protects cells from damage. Eating tomato sauce decreases the risk of developing many types of cancers.

Keep your blood pressure under control —. Hypertension (high blood pressure) ages your arteries and is responsible for heart attacks and strokes. Foods high in potassium are known to decrease blood pressure by five points; keeping your daily salt intake to only a teaspoon can take another three points off your blood pressure.

So, what do you think, have we had access to the fountain of youth all along?

Incorporate all of these things into your life for twelve weeks and then decide. Start an exercise program that you follow two to three times a week, substitute some of the unhealthy snack food you may be snacking on for grapes and nuts, cut back on the salt, eat potassium-rich foods like bananas, and enjoy a nice whole-wheat pasta dinner with tomato sauce!

Keep track of how you feel the day you start; write down how old you feel and things that bother you. Rate your energy level on a scale of one to ten. Every week, reevaluate how you are feeling. At the end of twelve weeks, see the difference; how old do you feel now? What is your energy level?

I believe that the fountain of youth is accessible to all of us. We just have to want it badly enough. How badly do you want it?

Are You Stressed??

Are you feeling like most of us these days—a little stressed? I have something that might help you get through it. EXERCISE! I know you probably find it hard to believe that exercise can help prevent diseases, boost your immune system, burn fat and build muscle, and relieve stress, too. But it can and it does.

The "magic" in exercise comes from three neuro-chemicals, serotonin, dopamine, and endorphins. Neurochemicals are chemicals that naturally occur in the nervous system and play a part in its functioning. Exercise helps increase neurochemicals, making us feel happier, less stressed.

Serotonin improves mood and helps to reduce depression. Serotonin can be decreased because of stress, anxiety, and a low-carbohydrate diet. Serotonin is elevated after a long run or workout, even at moderate intensity levels. With a rise in serotonin levels, you feel less stressed.

Dopamine can also be decreased by stress, anxiety, and a low-carbohydrate diet. Long periods of exercise at moderate intensity can elevate dopamine levels and make you feel happier.

Endorphins are often referred to as natural pain-killers. It is because of our endorphins that we have decreased pain while we exercise. Endorphins are responsible for the feeling of a "runner's high." The endorphin response to exercise increases with frequency of the exercise.

Any amount of exercise will have a positive effect on your mood. Activities that rely more on endurance than power create a rise in serotonin levels. The rise in serotonin that is experienced with moderate intensity exercise seems to be similar in nature to the rise in serotonin that we experience when we are with our good friends and family. When we engage in positive experiences, including exercise (yes, exercise is a positive experience) at low to moderate intensity levels, we see a rise in serotonin levels.

When serotonin levels rise, dopamine levels tend to rise as well. Endorphins respond to exercise regardless of the intensity of the workout. However, the more we exercise, the more endorphins we produce with each exercise.

Exercise boosts self-confidence. You can't not feel good about yourself after a good workout and the great sense of accomplishment it brings. Exercise relaxes tense muscles and can even help you sleep better. In this busy world, who can't use a good night of sleep?

I know, this a lot of information; the beauty is, you don't need to remember any of the names of these neuro-chemicals, and you don't need to understand how and why they make you feel better. You just have to give it a try and see for yourself. Pick the exercise of your choice, leave all your responsibilities behind for a little while, and do a little exercise.

You may be thinking, I am so overwhelmed as it is, how can I possibly fit in exercise? At first you will have to work really hard to fit in it, but once you begin, and start releasing those endorphins, serotonin, and dopamine, you will be looking forward to your next workout.

I can't think of a better way to step away from all the stress for a little while. Yes it will all still be waiting for you when you're done with your workout, but you'll be in a much better frame of mind to deal with it all.

Drink Up!

How much water are you drinking? We always hear how we need to drink eight 8-ounce glasses of water daily, but many of us don't know why we need so much water, so we don't drink that much. Although you would never be able to tell by our diets, water is actually more important than food. We can't go more than a few days without water, but we can go a couple of weeks without food (don't try it!).

On the average, 60 percent of our body is made of water. Our blood is about 90 percent water, our brain about 80 percent water, our muscles are about 75 percent water, our skin is 71 percent water, and bones are said to contain 22 percent water.

Many studies show that we need to consume eight 8-ounce glasses of water a day to replace the fluids lost through breathing, perspiration, urination, and bowel movements. Water is essential for digestion, improves blood pressure, and helps circulation, among other things.

With exercise, even more water is needed. Two hours before exercising, we should drink at least fourteen ounces of water. Gatorade did a study that showed that a well-hydrated person exercised 33 percent longer than a person who was not well-hydrated. The study also showed that half of the exercisers were dehydrated before they began to exercise.

Water assists in the contraction of our muscles. It's a shock absorber for bone and muscle. Additionally, water maintains your body temperature as it eliminates heat and rids our body of waste. When you don't get enough water, you dehydrate, and nothing functions as well as it should.

Fatigue can also be a side effect of dehydration, so if you find that you are constantly tired, try drinking more water. If you are not drinking enough water, the blood, brain, and muscles will suffer first because they have the highest percentage of water (and thus the highest need). Dehydration will affect your mental ability. Some studies have shown that as much as 95 percent of headaches are a side effect of dehydration, so before you take a pill to relieve your headache, try a glass of water. And remember that once you become thirsty, you have already begun to dehydrate.

If all these reasons aren't enough to get you drinking water, it also aids in weight loss! Water fills you up and may keep food cravings at bay by cleansing your palate. Water cleanses your palate by removing the taste of food from your mouth.

Water is inexpensive, readily accessible, and very important. If you're not a big fan of water, try putting some slices of orange, lemon, or lime in it. Iced tea and iced coffee are not substitutes for water. The caffeine in these drinks acts as a diuretic, which increases urination and speeds dehydration.

So, did you have your sixty-four ounces of water today? If not, there's no time like the present to get started drinking! (Water, that is!)

Chapter 3

Arm Yourself Against Illness

Genetics vs. Lifestyle

As we age, how much of our health is a result of genetics, and how much is a result of lifestyle? I think most of you will be surprised to learn that it's approximately an 80/20 split. Eighty percent of how we age is due to our lifestyle, while only 20 percent is genetically determined.

This is really great news! We now know that we have a lot more control of our health than previously believed. But with control comes responsibility—the responsibility to take care of your body. This control may begin very early in life, but if not, it's never to late to take responsibility and make healthier choices.

This is not to say that we should ignore our genetics. We need to be aware of our genetics as much as we can and work with them. Genetics doesn't mean you are destined to get a disease that runs in your family, but you should live your life in such a way that you may possibly avoid or minimize, to the best of your ability, the illnesses of your family.

Diet, exercise, avoiding toxins, using supplements wisely, getting enough sleep, decreasing stress, even acts of kindness—all are shown to diminish the effects of disease and aging. Exercise is known to be good for your heart, to lower blood pressure, and to promote weight loss, which can keep many illnesses at bay. Exercise also helps prevent osteoporosis, eliminates stress, may prevent cancer, promotes brain health, and much more.

A proper diet is a diet filled with nutrients. Nuts, fruits, vegetables, and whole grains can do wonders for your health. You are doing nothing to help your body fight the many diseases and illness we are at risk of when you eat cakes, cookies, and candy.

We have about 80 percent of the control—and we should all take advantage of that control. Every day that we don't take that control is a day that we can be getting closer to a serious illness. Thirty minutes of walking daily is said not only to prevent diseases, but to improve your health if you've already been diagnosed with an illness.

A diet high in antioxidants can do wonders. Antioxidants protect against free radicals, which are highly-reactive atoms or molecules which can cause cellular damage, impairing the immune system. These can contribute to many different diseases. Take advantage of the control: go for a walk, eat some berries, avoid toxins whenever possible, get a good night of sleep, and do something nice for someone. And hopefully you will be rewarded with good health, which ultimately means a good quality of life.

Childhood Obesity in America

The current generation of children is the first generation to have a lower life expectancy than their parents. This is thanks to the childhood obesity plaguing America. Over the past thirty years, childhood obesity has more than doubled. Obesity in children increases their risk of developing Type 2 diabetes as well as other serious chronic diseases.

Although having obese parents more than doubles a child's risk of being obese, it does not explain the increase in obesity over the past thirty years. So before we blame genetics, let's stop and ask ourselves: Are we doing everything we can to lower our children's weight and increase our children's life expectancy? If the answer is yes, we should be commended. If the answer is no, read on and see what we can do to help our children have healthier, happier lives today and tomorrow.

When it comes to making changes in our own lives, we need to take it one step at a time; and we have to do the same with our children. We don't want to overwhelm them. When I made the choice to change my pantry at home I did it a little at a time to give everyone a chance to adjust. Some members of my family adjusted, and some still complain about the whole-wheat bread and the natural peanut butter, but I'd rather that they complain about that than about the insulin needle that they will need if they should develop Type 2 diabetes.

Start by keeping a bowl of fresh fruits or vegetables on the counter. If it's out and easy to grab, the kids have a tendency to eat it without even being told to. My kids almost always eat whatever is in that bowl. It may be baby carrots, almonds, peaches, grapes, sliced cucumber, or sliced peppers. Give it a try—you might end up snacking on the fresh fruit and vegetables yourself.

For a great snack, try making your kids healthy shakes. They're simple to make, very healthy, and most kids love them. Just take fat-free milk (or 1 percent milk) and blend it with frozen fruits of your choice. Sometimes I add strawberries and blueberries, sometimes raspberries with mango, or I might add an apple or a banana. If you would rather use fresh fruit, just add a little ice to chill it. I find that adding a banana will thicken up the shake. Sometimes I even sneak in a little flaxseed. Flaxseed is a great natural way to lower cholesterol, lower blood pressure, and possibly prevent some cancers. You can't even taste the flaxseed in the shake. Fruit shakes are a great way to get your kids to eat a variety of fruits. You can even freeze the leftovers (if there are any) for a great frozen treat.

Make every attempt to keep partially hydrogenated oils out of kids' diets. You will find it in any peanut butter that is not natural, as well as in many cookies and in most margarine products. Start reading labels; it is imperative to all of us to have an idea of what is going into our bodies and our children's bodies.

We have to get our kids up and moving. Not every activity is for every child, but find what works for your child. My daughter plays Dance Dance Revolution (DDR) for hours at a time. It is a video game that she dances with. Maybe you'll find an activity that you can do with your child that will keep you both moving and create a special parent–child bond. Perhaps bowling is an activity that you can learn to enjoy together. Remember some of the great things we did when we were kids—the pogo stick, jump rope, the hula-hoop, and the Chinese jump rope? Try playing a game of hopscotch with your kids. You're only too old to do these things with your kids if you think you are. These are still so much fun and are a great way to burn those calories—at any age. Hey, you never know, you may find yourself on that pogo stick! I still find myself on it from time to time and when I wake up the next morning my burning quadriceps remind me of the fun I had with my kids the day before.

Cancer-Fighting Foods

It's upsetting how often we hear of another person getting cancer. We really need to fight against cancer; and with cancer everywhere, no one today can think that they are immune to the possibility of getting it. Start your fight against cancer today! Adding these foods to your diet will help you reduce your risk of cancer. We really need to be proactive. Let's all do our share to protect our health. If we don't take care of our bodies, who else will?

~Garlic helps in the fight against cancer of the esophagus, stomach, and colon.

~Avocados help fight free radicals; free-radical damage may lead to cancer and other diseases.

~Berries are filled with antioxidants, which prevent free radicals from forming. Berries can help prevent cancers from growing and spreading. I keep a bag of frozen mixed berries in the freezer at all times. Add them to a shake, put them over waffles, or add them to muffins.

~Tomatoes can help reduce the risk of prostate cancer. Tomatoes contain an antioxidant called lycopene, which is even more effective when ingested in cooked tomatoes. This makes tomato sauce and tomato soup especially healthy.

~Carrots, along with all the other vegetables that are high in beta-carotene, such as sweet potato, squash, and pumpkin, are high in antioxidants that help fight cancer.

~Cruciferous vegetables such as broccoli, cabbage, and cauliflower can protect you from free radicals that can damage the DNA of your cells. They also give protection against cancer-causing chemicals and may help slow down the growth of tumors.

~Green tea contains an ingredient called catechins which may not only reduce tumor cell growth but may also shrink tumors. Black tea also contains catechins, but green tea contains more.

~Whole grains contain antioxidants and fiber, which can help in the fight against colorectal cancer. Some whole-grain sources are brown rice, whole-wheat breads, whole oats, and whole-wheat pasta.

~Tumeric has an ingredient called curcumin (not cumin). According to the American Cancer Society, in lab studies curcumin has been shown to inhibit some kinds of cancer cells and to slow the spread of cancer or even shrink tumors.

~Green leafy vegetables contain antioxidants, beta-carotene, and lutein, which may limit the growth of some kinds of cancer cells.

~Grapes contain resveratrol and flavanoids, which are antioxidants that may aid in keeping cancer from spreading or even beginning. Studies have found that these antioxidants may limit the growth of many kinds of cancer cells.

~Beans are important in the cancer-fighting diet due to their high fiber content and high amounts of anti-oxidants. Add beans to your salads, or make a bean dip for your next party.

~Pineapples, apples, flaxseed, figs, grapefruit, papaya, and nuts are also said to help reduce the risk of cancer.

Now that you have some ammo against cancer, start using it. Sauté some garlic in tomato sauce and serve over whole-wheat pasta, add some broccoli and cauliflower serve some mixed berries for dessert with a cup of green tea and let the cancer cells be prepared for a battle!

Can You Lower Your Blood Pressure by Exercising?

By exercising regularly, you strengthen your muscles. Your heart is a muscle that gets stronger when you exercise it, just like any of your other muscles. A stronger heart will beat more efficiently. Your heart will pump more blood with less effort when it is stronger. So the answer to the question in the title is, Yes you can!

When your heart pumps more blood with less effort, the pressure on your arteries is decreased, and this results in lower blood pressure. By exercising, you will see a significant drop in your blood pressure. It may take one to three months before you see a drop in your blood pressure, but don't give up. Your blood pressure probably didn't increase overnight, so don't expect it to decrease overnight.

This drop in blood pressure may mean the difference between needing and not needing blood pressure medications. If you have ideal blood pressure, regular exercise may keep it from increasing as you age.

If you discontinue your exercise, you can expect your blood pressure to rise to pre-exercise numbers; it will only decrease for as long as you continue to exercise. If you lose weight as a result of exercise, your blood pressure will probably stay lower due to the loss of weight. But chances are that if you stop exercising, you will put the weight back on.

All exercise is important for different reasons, but when we are focusing on blood pressure, aerobic exercises are where you want to spend your time. The idea is to get your heart rate up. Walking, jogging, jumping rope (with or without a rope), running up and down the stairs, riding a bike, and so forth, are all great aerobic activities. Even activities such as raking leaves, shoveling snow, and vacuuming will help. If the activity raises your heart rate, it can help your blood pressure.

Try to work in thirty minutes of aerobic activity on as many days as you can. It does not have to be thirty minutes straight; ten minutes here and ten minutes there—it all adds up to a healthier heart, which means lower blood pressure. I know life is hectic; it's so much easier to take blood pressure medicine then it is to get thirty minutes of physical activity. If time really isn't on your side, just remember that something is better than nothing! Start with even as little as five minutes daily, everyone has five minutes. You will feel so good from the five minutes that it will become ten minutes, and so on.

In addition to exercise, watching your sodium intake, maintaining a healthy weight, eating a healthy diet, and limiting alcohol intake all can help decrease high blood pressure. Also, be sure to follow your doctor's orders when it comes to taking blood pressure medicines.

Osteoporosis: Are You protecting Yourself?

Osteoporosis is a condition that causes the bones to become thin and brittle, which makes them susceptible to breaks and fractures. The disease has been termed the "silent epidemic" since there are no symptoms or warning signs prior to a fracture. Although both men and woman are at risk of developing osteoporosis, it is more common in women and the risk increases with age, even more so after menopause. However, there are steps that can be taken at any age to minimize the chances of getting this condition. Osteoporosis is a preventable disease.

Bones provide support for your body and allow you to move. They are living organs that help protect your heart, lungs, and brain from injury. Your bones store vital minerals. When you have osteoporosis your bones lose some of these minerals, which is what makes them fragile and more likely to break or fracture.

Exercising may lower your risk of developing osteoporosis. The National Osteoporosis Society recommends exercising at least three times per week, for a minimum of twenty minutes each time. Exercise can slow bone mineral loss. Exercise is also important because muscle pulling on bone builds denser, stronger bones. If you have already been diagnosed with osteoporosis you should consult with your physician to discuss limitations before beginning your exercise program.

Weight-bearing exercises and weight-training exercises are both very important aspects of your workout program. A weight-bearing exercise is any exercise that uses your bones for support. This includes brisk walking, jogging, stair climbing, using the tread climber, etc. Weight-training exercise is any exercise that involves resistance, such as free weights, exercise machines, resistance bands, etc.

In addition to regular exercise, diet is also very important for bone health. If you are deficient in vitamin B12, you are at greater risk of developing osteoporosis. Fruits and vegetables help to protect our skeletons, while a diet high in salt and fat can drain our bones of calcium. Calcium is the most important nutrient for attaining peak bone mass and for preventing and treating this condition. Calcium strengthens your bones. Vitamin D is also very important in assisting the body in its absorption of calcium. Milk contains a lot of calcium in a form that the body can easily absorb. So skip the soda and grab a glass of low-fat or fat-free milk.

Make the choice today to begin protecting those very important bones that support your very precious body.

Balance and Aging

How is your balance? Did you know that falls are one of the leading causes of injury-related deaths   and hospitalization in people aged sixty-five years and older? Often falls are due to a lack of balance. People lose their balance with age, usually due to inactivity. With balance, it's use it or lose it. So let's start using it!

Balance is a skill. The ability to control and maintain the body's position as it moves through space is a skill which, with practice, you can develop and maintain. You can also build and maintain a strong core. If you don't exercise to maintain and improve your balance, you will lose it.

Balance depends upon vision, information from the inner ear, and proprioception—the ability to sense the position, location, orientation, and movement of the body and its parts.

All these senses work together. Proprioception is used when you close your eyes and lift your arm and still know which way your palm is turned. It tells you where you are and where you belong in space. Decreased proprioception, hearing, and vision all play a role in the deterioration of balance.

Exercise is important to maintaining and even improving balance. Start by standing on one foot for ten seconds, then switch to the other foot. In a few days, try holding it for fifteen seconds, and gradually add more time. The use of a balance board is great for balance. Exercising with a yoga ball instead of a bench can also improve balance.

Our abdominal and lower back muscles play a large part in controlling posture and balance. Therefore a strong core will improve both balance and posture.

Don't become a statistic when you are sixty-five. Sit up straight, strengthen your abdominals and back, and do some balancing exercises. It might just keep you from visiting the emergency room with a broken bone. And you are never too old to start, just take it slow. If you haven't exercised in a long time, have a friend spot you to avoid injury; and always practice caution when doing any balancing exercises.

Exercising: It's a Quality of Life Issue

When your health is good, life is just better. When your health suffers, nothing is quite as pleasurable as it was. Take the common cold, for example. Look at how the quality of your life diminishes just from having a head cold. You know it's going to pass within a week, but boy, is it a long week.

Many illnesses don't pass within a week and can diminish the quality of your life indefinitely. Don't be the one to stand in the way of your best quality of life. Make the decision to live the healthiest life you are capable of living. Good health can dramatically improve the quality of your life.

Some of the Benefits of Exercising

- Decrease in Blood Pressure	- Increase in Muscle Mass
- Decreased Risk of Stroke	- Decreased Risk of Osteoporosis
- Increase in Metabolism	-Improves Sleep
- Decreased Risk of Diabetes	-Decreased Risk of Heart Disease
- Reduces the Risk of Colon Cancer	- Decrease in Cholesterol
- Reduces Depression and Anxiety	- Decrease in Body Fat

Promotes Psychological Well Being

It is important to remember that health improvements take effect sooner than improvements in fitness and endurance. Improvements in fitness usually occur with less training than that required for weight loss. So if you don't immediately see the change in your body on the outside, don't give up because there are great changes going on inside. You will start seeing changes on the outside before you know it. Don't give up—and be sure to think before you eat! Make sure what you eat is as good for your body as what you do. The combination is really amazing.

General Guidelines for Resistance Training

In order for our bodies to change, we need to give it a reason. The muscle needs to be challenged and fatigued in order to see results—but never in pain. It is good to feel the burn, but *not* to feel the pain.

When you begin any new exercise, it is important not to overload the muscle. The fact that the body is getting adjusted to a new exercise is enough of a stimulus. Do not work to the point of fatigue the first time you do any new exercise.

After your first few workouts, you do want to get your muscle fatigued. If you are not fatigued, you need to increase your resistance, or increase the repetitions in the exercise.

You must maintain control of your movement during the entire exercise. You control your resistance; don't let your resistance control you.

It is important not to over-train. Muscles generally need forty-eight hours to recover. Do not work out every day. Our muscles grow when they rest.

One hour is an ideal workout time.

Change your workouts. A slightly different stimulus will increase the variety of muscles recruited. Your muscles get used to the same routine and therefore are not challenged. Change it up regularly by changing the order, the weight, the exercise, the angle of the handgrip, or mix free weights, bands, and machines.

Chapter 4

If You're Going to Exercise, Make It Count

Strength

10 Reasons Why You Should be Weight Training

Yes, you! Strength training is important for both men and women. Here's why...

1. **Stop Muscle Loss** — Adults who do not strength-train may lose up to 1 percent of muscle mass annually. At the end of ten years, that is a 10 percent loss of muscle mass. This decrease in muscle begins in our thirties. Strength training helps maintain muscle mass and increases our physical ability, which reduces the chance of injury and improves our self-confidence.

2. **Avoid Decrease in Metabolism** — Our metabolism doesn't slow down just because we are forty or fifty years old, it slows down as we lose our muscle mass. Muscle is a very active tissue and when it decreases, our metabolism slows. The average adult has a 2 to 5 percent decrease in metabolism every ten years, according to William Evans and Irving Rosenberg (*Biomarkers,*1992). If you start rebuilding that muscle, you will begin to increase your metabolism.

3. **Reduce Body Fat** — Increasing muscle mass will increase your appetite slightly. It is really important that when your appetite increases you make healthy choices about adding calories to your diet. If you reach for cookies and candy after your workout, you are not going to see the results you were hoping for.

4. **Decrease Your Risk of Osteoporosis** — Creating stress on your bones during weight training can increase your bone density. As a result, you can reduce your risk of developing osteoporosis.

5. **Reduce the Risk of Diabetes** — Strength training can improve insulin sensitivity and improve glucose tolerance.

6. **Improve Posture** — Strength training improves posture, which can help to eliminate neck and back pain. An added benefit is a taller appearance.

7. **Reduce Blood Pressure**—Studies show that strength training may reduce resting blood pressure. However, a combination of strength training and cardiovascular training is even more effective in lowering blood pressure.

8. **Reduce Risk of Back Injuries** — Lower back muscles are at increased risk of injury when they are weaker. A study showed that after ten weeks of strength training targeting the back, patients had less back pain. My clients often tell me how good the back exercises feel as they are performing them.

9. **Reduce Arthritic Pain** — Strong muscles act as shock absorbers for the joints while they support and protect joints affected by arthritis. Muscles can take pressure off the joints, thus alleviating some of the pain that comes from arthritis.

10. **Look Better, Feel Better** — Strength training will help you look better, feel better, and function better. Ultimately you will *be* better.

Weight training can and should be done at any age. Just start off with light weights and be sure that your form is correct, to avoid injuries—and take it slow! Finding the fountain of youth may seem impossible and the "battle of the bulge" may seem like a losing battle as we get older. However, with hard work and determination you can win these battles and slow down the aging process. Start a weight-training program today and you will look and feel better before you know it. You didn't gain the weight and lose the muscle overnight so you won't gain the muscle and lose the fat overnight. Be patient, and more important, be determined. You are worth it.

Give yourself an incentive to begin. After one month on your new exercise program treat yourself to a massage or a manicure to reward yourself for all your hard work. It takes a lot of determination to take that first step. I know you have it in you!

Getting Fit with Little Ones

I know it is difficult to do any kind of exercise when you have little ones, but it's not impossible. Here are some great ideas to help you get in shape while cooking dinner, doing laundry, and playing with your children. This exercise routine is excuse-proof.

Start jumping rope, it tones the entire body and is one of the most efficient workouts. Yes, you probably will look spastic when you first start, but your body will look awesome in no time. Your kids will be thrilled to be playing with you and you'll be setting a great fitness example for them.

Buy an adult hula hoop and start hula-hooping. Hula-hooping targets your abdominal muscles, hips, and waistline. It is a great cardio and strength workout. You may burn as many as 100 calories in just ten minutes. No, you are not too old and no, you don't need to be any good at it to get killer abs! Just keep going, squeeze those abs each time you try and when you miss (which will be often for most of us) squat to pick up the hula hoop and get an additional workout on your legs and buttocks. Go to www.sports-hoop.com for more information on hula hoops.

While putting your laundry away, run up and down the stairs. Then try taking it two steps at a time. When you've mastered that, try going up backwards to work different muscles in your legs. It's great for your heart and lungs and you'll look great in those short-shorts before you know it.

Dance while you clean. You have to clean anyway, so put on some great music and start dancing off those pounds while you're sweeping up the spilled Cheerios or wiping all those little fingerprints off the appliances.

When you have to get up because the children are bickering, get up from the chair s-l-o-w-l-y, then sit back down s-l-o-w-l-y, then get up—it's a great lower body exercise. And maybe by the time you get up, the kids will have worked out their spat on their own.

While you're cooking your low-fat dinner, squeeze your abs and hold for ten seconds. Do that for eight reps to start with and work your way up to fifteen. Doing that may also keep your mind off of picking while you cook. While eating your dinner, squeeze your gluteus maximus (glutes) and hold for ten seconds. Do that for eight reps to start with, and work your way up to fifteen.

Studies show that ten minutes of aerobic exercise is about all you need to produce enough endorphins to make you feel good. So not only will you look fabulous, but you will feel fabulous, which will give you more patience to deal with all the challenges the day has in store for you.

You will be surprised at how quickly your strength and endurance will improve. Don't get discouraged if you can't hula-hoop or jump rope well; unless you are entering a contest, no one cares. But everyone will be impressed with how great you'll look. It's a cheap, easy, challenging, and fun workout that you can do with your kids, or while doing your chores. So what are you waiting for, go have some fun with your kids and get in shape!

More Great Exercises for You and Your Little Ones

The yoga ball is another very effective yet inexpensive tool to help you get in shape while bonding with your children. Get a Hippity Hop ball for your little ones so they can play, too.

<u>SQUAT</u>

-Stand with a yoga ball between your lower back and the wall

-Walk your feet forward about a foot; keep your arms by your side

-Squeeze abs and slowly bend knees; do not let your knee go past your toe line, and do not let your hip go below your knee

-Slowly return to starting position

<u>CRUNCH</u>

-Lie on the ball with the ball placed under your lower back. Your head and shoulders should not be on the ball (For extra support, try putting your toes against the wall while placed firmly on the ground)

-Place hands behind your head but don't lock your fingers together; keep your head in a neutral position

-While holding your abs in, slowly lift toward the ceiling, being careful not to bend your neck

-Slowly return to starting position

REVERSE CRUNCH

-Lie face up on the floor with the ball between your bent legs; squeeze the ball tightly and dig your heels in to hold in place

-Place hands behind head without locking fingers. Bring your knees in toward your chest, lifting your hips slightly off the floor

-Slowly return hips to the floor, trying to keep abs contracted throughout

WALL PRESS

-Position ball against the wall, face ball with hands a shoulder-width apart, straight in front of you without locking your elbows, holding the ball in place

-Slowly bend elbow and lean into the ball as your heels lift off the floor

-Slowly return to starting position

Make it a game for your little ones: Have them run under the ball when you are in the starting position;

they can pretend it's a bridge and they have to be out before you lean in

BALL BRIDGE

-Lie face up on the ball with neck and back supported by the ball

-Bend knees and keep feet hip-distance apart, keeping your body straight from your head to your knees

-Slowly squeeze buttocks up

-Slowly lower and return to starting position

Here's another bridge for the kids: make sure you keep your buttocks up or the kids will get "trapped" under the bridge

BALL LIFT

-Stand with your feet hip-distance apart, holding your yoga ball behind you

-Squeeze your shoulder blades together and hold abs in

-Raise the ball *slowly* away from you while keeping your arms straight, but not locked

-Slowly return to starting position

BALL SQUEEZE

-Straddle the ball between your legs with feet positioned behind the ball

-Squeeze the ball and hold for a count of eight

-Slowly release and repeat

-Have your little ones count with you

SINGLE-LEG HIP LIFT

-Lie on the floor on your back with knees bent and heels pressed into the ball, which is in front of you

-Keep arms to the side

-Keep your left leg on the ball and slowly straighten your right leg, extending it toward the ceiling, bringing your hips and back off the floor

-Slowly return to starting position

-Repeat with your right leg

SHOULDER PRESS

-Grab a couple of cans of vegetables or baby formula

-Sit on your ball with feet shoulder-width apart

-Bring arms up in line with your shoulders and bend elbows so that your elbow makes a right angle with your arm. Fists should be facing the ceiling

-Lift the cans slowly up and out, not directly over your spine but over your forehead, straightening your arms without locking your elbows

-Slowly return to starting position

-Repeat

For best results, each of these exercises should be performed in a slow and controlled manner. Don't rush it, the quality is more important than the quantity. Your muscles can't count but they do know when you're doing a quality move and so will everyone else.

So what are you waiting for, your not thinking of an excuse are you????

10 Tips to a Rockin' Workout

1. Variety is essential to a great workout. Muscles have memory; they need to be constantly challenged in order to change. Variations may include changing the resistance used (dumbbell, barbell, exercise bands, etc.), changing the intensity, the amount of weight used, or even changing your hand or leg placement.

2. Take it slowly. Gradual progression is important and will reduce your risk of injury.

3. Muscles grow when they rest. It is important to allow yourself at least forty-eight hours before working the same muscle group again.

4. Never use momentum; your movements should be slow and controlled throughout the entire exercise. If you use momentum or speed, you will greatly increase your risk of injury.

5. Move only the joint or joints necessary to perform the movement; for example, when performing a bicep curl, the only joint used is the elbow. Keep the shoulder stable throughout the entire exercise.

6. After approximately ninety minutes of working out, you run the risk of over-training. Exercise bolsters your immune system, but over-training will weaken it. You may also increase your risk of

injury. Don't expect to transform your body in just one workout. Be patient.

7. Muscles weigh three times as much as fat, so although you may be losing fat, as you gain lean muscle the numbers on the scale may not go down, the may even go up a bit. Let your clothing, not the scale, be the judge.

8. When doing aerobics, it is beneficial to use a heart monitor to track your training heart rate. To figure out your maximal heart rate, see chapter 5.

9. Variety is essential in your aerobic workout as well. You can change your speed, increase and decrease the incline, work with hands or without hands. Try jumping rope for variety one day and taking a brisk walk another. It doesn't matter how you change it up, just be sure to change it up.

10. Make it fun, grab a friend, put on your favorite music—exercise really can be fun and it will make you look great and feel great.

What to Look For When Choosing a Personal Trainer

When warm weather comes will you be ready for your shorts and tank top? I know you probably started thinking about it by now, but have you started doing anything to prepare for that summer wardrobe yet?

If you know you have some work to do before putting on those summer clothes, but can't seem to get motivated, maybe it's time to seek the help of a personal trainer. Here are some things to consider when choosing one.

You are going to be working very closely with this person, so it is important that you feel comfortable around him or her. You need to be motivated and inspired by the person you are trusting to help you be the best you that you can be.

It is important that your trainer's priorities are the same as yours. For some people it's just about results, while for others it's about a whole lifestyle.

Does the trainer practice what he or she preaches? It is very difficult to be motivated by a trainer who is not walking the walk.

Can you afford it? If it's really stretching your budget, you may not be able to stay with it for long. Find out about group training. You get much of the same benefits of private sessions at as little as a third of the cost.

If you have injuries, will the trainer work around them? As we age, we all have one injury or another. It's no excuse for not working out. Exercise can often be helpful for certain injuries.

Is the atmosphere in which you'll work out one that you will feel comfortable in? Some people thrive in the gym atmosphere while others like a more private setting.

Is safety the first priority? If the exercise isn't done in the safest manner, you are more likely to become injured.

Choose someone who really cares about your success. If you feel like your trainer is only in it for the money, you probably will not go as far as you are capable of going. Your success should also be your trainers success.

Make sure the person is certified. Not all personal trainers are certified.

Can You Do Too Much of a Good Thing?

Yes, you can. Exercise is great, but you can do too much of it and then it is called over-training. This is when the volume and intensity of an individual's exercise exceeds the person's recovery capacity, at which point progress stops. You may even begin to lose strength. You can over-train by pushing your body to do too much. Over-training might be achieved by working out for too long, working out too often, working out with too much intensity, or by not resting when your body needs rest. Listen to your body.

Our muscles grow and strengthen while they rest. It is counterproductive to work the same muscles two days in a row. Depending on the intensity of a workout, your body needs approximately forty-eight hours rest before working the same body parts. After a really intense workout you may need even more resting time.

Exercising does a lot of great things for you. It gives you strength, energy, helps you sleep, and puts you in a good mood. Over-training can do the complete opposite.

Symptoms of over-training may include:

Elevated resting heart rate   Increased susceptibility to infections

Increased chance of injury   Irritability

Fatigue	Depression
Persistent muscle soreness	Insomnia

You will know if you have overdone it if ten to fifteen minutes after you stop exercising you are still out of breath; two hours after the exercise you feel unusually tired; you can't sleep well that night or the following night; or your resting heart rate increased by 10 percent or more.

If you suspect that you are over-training, take some time off and let your muscles rest and recover. The longer you have been over-training, the more time you will need to rest and recover. It is okay to strength train every day, just not the same muscles every day. Make a schedule—perhaps do legs and abs on Monday, Wednesday, and Friday and work arms and back on Tuesday and Thursday, and give yourself some time off on the weekend.

It is also very important to increase weight in a slow and controlled way. Don't go suddenly from using three-pound dumbbells for your bicep curls to eight-pound dumbbells. Make it a gradual increase.

As you become more fit, you still need the same rest and recovery time, if not more, because you will be doing more. Make sure you are getting proper nutrition and proper sleep to help you recover from your workouts.

Keeping a workout log is the most effective way to keep track of your workout. You can track how much weight you used and which body parts you worked.

Although I have really focused on strength training, you can also over-train during your cardio workout if you work out intensely. If you are running, you might want to take a couple of days off and walk or ride a bike instead to help avoid injuries. If you are new to running it is advisable to start slowly and work your way up. Start with a jog and slowly increase your speed and duration. It is okay to do cardio every day, but not advisable to do high-intensity cardio daily.

Exercise is great, but if it is not done with caution, it can be a very harmful thing for you. After all, too much of a good thing is still too much.

Being Fit vs. Being Athletic

Being physically fit and being athletic are two different things. People are often surprised to hear that I am not athletic at all. I don't want a small ball, a big ball, a hard ball, or a soft ball thrown at me or to me. I don't want to race anyone around a track. I don't want to hit a ball with a bat or a stick. I don't even want to hit a puck or try to get a ball into a basket. I have no desire to compete against anyone in any sport.

But I love a great workout. I enjoy running around a track or jogging on the treadmill. I love working with a medicine ball and a yoga ball. I enjoy the victory of beating my best record on the elliptical or on the exercise bike. I love the feeling of getting stronger and improving my endurance. I get excited each time I improve my balance and my coordination.

The definition of fitness is "a measure of the body's ability to function efficiently and effectively in work and leisure activities, to be healthy, to resist hypokinetic diseases [conditions that occur from a sedentary lifestyle], and to meet emergency situations." Fitness makes you feel better and gives you the strength and energy you need to get through the day. Being fit may help prevent or fight off many diseases.

The definition of an athlete is a person who participates regularly in a sport. An athlete's goal revolves around the specific sport that he or she is playing.

Just because you are not athletic doesn't mean you should not start an exercise program. And starting an exercise program doesn't mean you have to consider running a marathon! Running a marathon is not necessarily an outcome of being fit. Someone training for a marathon has entirely different goals than a person who is training for fitness.

Even if you have never thrown, caught, rolled, or kicked a ball in your life, you can still be a fit person—or become a fit person—with a bit of hard work, proper training, and some discipline.

There's really no excuse. Just about anyone can take a brisk walk, which may turn into a jog, which may turn into running. Never say never. Most anyone can do bicep curls; just start with a light weight and watch how in no time you will be increasing the weights. Nearly anyone can do a couple of squats which eventually will become a full set of squats. Practice you balance; at first you may be disappointed with your balancing skills, but before you know it you will be balancing a little longer, and then a lot longer. If you stick with your fitness training, in no time you can be fit.

The Importance of Stretching

Stretching is a very important component of fitness. Stretching helps improve flexibility, but stretching can do much more than that. Stretching can reduce your chance of exercise-related injuries to joints, muscles, and tendons; improve posture; help with mental and physical relaxation; reduce muscle soreness; relieve symptoms of PMS; and enhance overall fitness. Although stretching can be very beneficial, if it is not done correctly, you do risk injury. Stretching is important for the very active and the not-so active. Just sitting at a desk all day can make you stiff. Stretching can help relieve some of that stiffness.

Before we begin, though, here are some things to avoid when stretching:

One common mistake is stretching at the beginning of a workout. It is important to warm up before stretching. Stretching cold muscles increases your chance of injuring them. Muscles are like rubber bands; if you put a rubber band in the refrigerator for a little while and then try to stretch it, it will be a bit stiff. Now take that same rubber band and rub it to warm it up—now stretch it. The warm rubber band stretches much more easily. That's the difference between stretching warm muscles and cold muscles. *A warm-up should be at least five minutes long and raise your body's temperature.* This could be done with walking, jumping jacks, knee lifts, marching in place, etc.

Another mistake is stretching until you're in pain. A little discomfort is okay, but you don't want to be in pain, you just want to feel the muscles pulling. Little by little you will be able to go further into your stretch. Don't rush it.

Don't bounce while stretching; bouncing will increase the risk of injury.

Don't hold your breath while stretching; steady breathing is very important during all kinds of exercise.

Here are some tips for a great stretch:

Hold each stretch for about ten to thirty seconds.

If you don't have time to warm up before your stretch, try a few stretches when you step out of a warm bath or shower. The warm water elevates the body's core temperature enough to make the muscles more pliable, reducing risk of injury.

Some people are more flexible than others. Genetics, gender, and age all play a role in how flexible one might be. As we age we tend to lose some flexibility, but don't worry, flexibility can improve with regular training. Like anything else, you just need to stick with it.

Just recently I incorporated stretching into my regular workout. I was doing it sporadically until I realized that my recovery was much quicker when I stretched. I was always too busy to take the time to stretch before but I now realize that my workouts are actually better because I am not as sore and tight.

So take a few minutes and stretch: it feels good, it's relaxing and it is so good for you!

Chapter 5

If You're Going to Exercise, Make It Count

Cardio

Are You Getting the Most Out of Your Cardio Workout?

In order to answer that question, wear a heart monitor during your cardiovascular workout. In order to tell if you are getting the maximum benefit from your workout, you need to gauge just how hard you are working. My motto is "If you're going to do it, make it count." Knowing what your heart rate is during your workout can let you know how well you are working toward your goal.

A few years ago my husband and I were on vacation in Bermuda. While we were there, we used the gym in our hotel. A woman came into the gym and was using the treadmill. She was walking at a very comfortable pace the entire time she was on the treadmill. It was an ideal pace for a warm-up or a cool-down but it would not have been very effective if her intention was to lose weight or improve her endurance.

I felt badly for the woman. It takes a lot of motivation and discipline to be in the gym on a beautiful day in Bermuda; but she didn't have all the necessary information to make it count. Don't get me wrong, what she was doing was much better for her than sipping a pina colada on the beach but she probably was not making any progress toward the goal she was striving for.

Before you begin your cardio routine, you need to figure out what your maximal heart rate (MHR) is. There are two different methods for figuring out your MHR.

The straight-line method is simple. Just take 220 and subtract your age from it. This method is not completely accurate since every person who is the same age is not at the same fitness level, but it is an excellent guideline.

After you have determined your MHR using the straight-line method you can figure out how high your heart rate should be.

These are the guidelines:

60–70 percent of your MHR burns fat.

70–80 percent of your MHR improves your cardiovascular and respiratory systems. This is great for endurance and burns even more calories.

For most people, it is not necessary to work above 80 percent of your MHR.

The second formula is the Karvonen method and is more accurate. First you need to know your resting heart rate. The best time to get this is when you first wake up in the morning. The formula is 220 minus your age, minus your resting heart rate (RHR), times desired exertion plus your resting heart rate.

Here are examples using both methods for a thirty-year-old person:

Straight line 220 – 30 (age) = 190

190 x 75 percent = 142.5

142.5 is a good heart rate if you are looking to burn fat and improve cardiovascular and respiratory systems for the average thirty-year-old.

Karvonen formula 220 – 30 (age) – 65 (RHR) x 75 percent (great for endurance) + 65 (RHR) =158.75

158.75 would be ideal for a thirty-year-old with a resting heart rate of 65.

Using the Karvonen formula almost always comes out higher than the straight-line method.

I know it seems a little complicated, but it is important information. If you're going to spend your time doing cardio, you want your workout to be as effective as possible. As you continue to work out you will have to increase your workout intensity in order to keep your heart rate up. Walking at a 3.0 on the treadmill may bring your heart rate up for the present, but if you stick with it, in no time you will need to increase to a 3.5 or maybe a 4.0 in order to get your heart rate up. The more advanced you are, the more you'll have to do to get your heart rate up. Be sure to start each workout with a warm-up. It's also very important to bring your heart rate back down before your complete your workout. Drink lots of water; if you are working to "make it count" you will definitely need lots water.

Benefits of Interval Training

Interval training is a very simple concept with a lot of benefits. The concept is basically to go fast, then go slow, then repeat. This alternates periods of high intensity with periods of low intensity.

Most everyone can do interval training. Interval training can be performed on almost any cardiovascular machine, treadmill, stair climber, exercise bike, elliptical, etc. You do not need machines to do interval training, it can also be performed by bicycling, swimming, or running.

These higher and lower intensity periods are repeated several times to form a complete workout. Often, people spend their workout performing continuous training exercises. These are exercises in which the intensity level is kept the same throughout the workout. For example, walking at 3.5 miles per hour at a zero percent incline for twenty-five minutes. Continuous training is very effective, but it is to your benefit to change up your routine by combining continuous training and interval training.

Interval training can help you improve cardiovascular fitness, increase speed, improve overall aerobic capability, burn more calories, increase your workout duration, and reach new exercise levels. Interval training is beneficial for exercisers at all levels.

To start, choose an exercise that you enjoy, such as walking, jogging, swimming, or biking. Next, determine your lower-intensity level. This is usually 50–65 percent target heart rate. Then increase the intensity level to where you feel like you are working hard to very hard (depending on your fitness level) but avoid reaching a level over 85 percent target heart rate. It would be beneficial to use a heart rate monitor for interval training. (See above, "Are you getting the most out of your cardio workout?" to calculate your target heart rate.)

You may change your speed randomly or choose a period of high intensity for one minute and low intensity for two minutes, and keep repeating. To increase your intensity, you can increase your speed, increase the incline, or start using your arms. In your next workout you can change the ratio; your workout can be different every time, which will keep you from becoming bored.

Interval training can be very helpful if you are trying a new exercise. If you were a beginner jogger, it would be very difficult to jog continuously without first building up to it; you will probably fatigue quickly and even give up. However, if you begin with intervals of walking with intervals of jogging, the workout will be much more enjoyable and effective.

Sample Interval Training Workout:

A warm-up followed by a good stretch is recommended before beginning your workout

Five minutes of low-intensity work, for example, walking

Two to three minutes of higher-intensity work. Reach your target heart zone by walking faster, jogging, increasing the incline, or swinging your arms. Remember to keep your heart rate below 85 percent of your target heart rate

Five minutes of low-intensity work—slow down

Two to three minutes of high-intensity work—reach your target heart zone again

Five minutes of low-intensity work

Five minutes to cool down

Go ahead, give it a try! The only thing you have to lose is a little weight.

So You Don't Run?

Well, don't worry, neither did I. The most running I ever did was to the mailbox and back on a cold day. Now I really enjoy it. I love the way it makes me feel. I look forward to getting on the treadmill and running. I have discovered for myself what a runner's high feels like.

I was about thirty-nine when I started. First I was just walking on the treadmill, then I went to a slow jog, then I moved to a faster jog, and now I am running. If anyone had told me that I'd ever run, I'd have said they were crazy, and yet here I am, not only running but also loving it. You can start running at any age.

Just start slowly. You really do have to walk before you can run. You may be wondering why you should run, and I used to wonder the same thing. Here are some reasons that might motivate you to give it a try.

-Running helps lower blood pressure by maintaining the elasticity of the arteries. When you run, your arteries expand and contract more than usual, helping keep the arteries elastic and the blood pressure low.

-Running helps maximize the lungs' potential. Deep breaths force the lungs to use more tissue. Fifty percent of lung tissue which is normally not used, gets used during running.

-Running strengthens the heart and may help prevent heart attacks. The heart of an inactive person beats 36,000 more times each day than the heart of a runner.

-Because running helps the body function better generally, improved sleep is a benefit.

-Running is one of the top aerobic activities for weight loss.

-Running prevents the muscle and bone loss associated with osteoporosis.

And of course there is the runner's high, which is a mild euphoria that comes during (and after) running.

What more can you ask for?

Don't Forget to Breathe

I know you're probably thinking, How can I forget to breathe? But often during the intensity of exercise people *do* forget to breathe and even have a tendency to hold their breath. Holding your breath during exercise can be dangerous. The body needs oxygen and when you hold your breath, you are not taking in any oxygen, so the heart has to work harder to pump the blood to deliver what oxygen you have. *This increases your heart rate and may be dangerous.* If you have high blood pressure, it can be even more dangerous. Breathing also releases carbon dioxide, which can't be expelled when you hold your breath. Every cell in our body needs oxygen to produce energy. Holding your breath can make you dizzy, nauseous, or disoriented.

I know it seems like just another thing to concentrate on while you're exercising. But it is as important as your form and your timing when it comes to having a safe and effective workout.

I find that if I count out loud while I am doing my weight training, it forces me to exhale with every repetition. You can't say, "One, two, three," without inhaling and exhaling. I recommend you exhale on the exertion, which is generally the harder part of the exercise, and inhale on the "rest," but if the reverse works better for you, that's fine. Just don't forget to breathe!

During cardio, breathing should be deep and strong, not shallow. You should develop a smooth, steady, and consistent breathing pattern. Breathing shouldn't be so much work, should it? But like I tell my clients all the time, I don't make the rules, I just enforce them.

Feel Ten Years Younger by Walking

As we age, our aerobic capacity decreases. Aerobic capacity is defined as the maximum amount of oxygen the body can use during a specified period, usually during intense exercise. Decreased aerobic capacity decreases our energy over time. However, walking on a regular basis can increase your aerobic capacity enough to make you feel as much as ten years younger. In addition, walking can:

Reduce cardiovascular disease by as much as 30 to 50 percent

Decrease osteoarthritis pain and improve stability, endurance, and agility

Lower blood pressure and reduce the risk of heart attack

Help reduce sleep problems

Reduce risk of dementia

Decrease depression and anxiety

Decrease the incidence of cancer, stroke, and diabetes

Strengthen muscles, bones, and joints

Improve mental health

In addition, walking will increase the number of calories you burn each day and can increase your muscle mass, which helps your body burn more calories throughout the day—not just while you are exercising but while you are resting as well.

Studies show that thirty to sixty minutes of daily walking is ideal for most of us, and while that may seem like a lot, the good news is that *any* amount of walking is beneficial. The key is to just get up and get started.

If you are finding it impossible to get in even twenty minutes of walking on a regular basis, start with ten minutes a day, and aim for at least three days a week. If finding even ten minutes is nearly impossible, try the basics, such as taking the stairs instead of the elevator, or parking further away from your destination. I have a client who would walk through the front door to go around to the backyard, just to get a little extra walking in. I have other clients who walk on their lunch breaks. It all adds up.

If you look hard enough, you can find ten minutes three times a week. Once you get started and begin feeling the benefits, you will want to start adding to it and all the excuses that were there will start to diminish. Then thirty minutes won't seem so overwhelming. You might even start to look forward to it.

Grab a friend, grab your iPod, or just enjoy some quiet alone time. You will feel better and look better.

How to Get the Most Out of Your Walk

We've said that walking on a regular basis can make you feel up to ten years younger. It can also help you burn more calories throughout the day. With that in mind, I'm sure you're anxious to start walking.

Start with a warm-up — Warm up by walking at a comfortable pace for about five minutes.

Stretch — Stretch your hamstrings, quads, and calf muscles before you begin.

Use proper posture — Look in front of you, keep your arms at ninety degrees, keep your abs and buttocks tight, and keep shoulders relaxed.

Push off with your toes and land on your heels.

For beginners, walk at a fast enough pace that your breathing is increased without making you feel breathless.

Don't use ankle weights or hand weights. When using weights you increase your risk of back injury, torn ligaments and muscle strain. I feel that the risk of injury outweighs the benefits.

Buy a pedometer. Guidelines suggest that we take 10,000 steps a day. How many steps are you walking? A sedentary person walks 1,000–3,000 steps daily. If that is you, start by trying to add on at least fifty steps every day until you get up to the recommended amount to benefit your health.

Join a walking club. Some malls have walking clubs, or you can start one yourself, you might just be doing your friends a big favor by taking the first "step," after which you can all get started together.

You will feel so good about walking and also about helping a friend. Invest in a decent pair of sneakers; your feet will thank you. Your sneakers should be one half to one size bigger than what you usually wear because your feet are likely to swell.

Drink water before, during, and after your walk.

Swinging your arms increases the intensity of your walk. I know it looks a little silly (my kids laugh at me when I do it) but it's worth being the brunt of a few giggles to make the most out of your walk.

Cool down for a few minutes by going back to that comfortable pace that you started with. Finish off with another stretch and some more water.

Do whatever it takes to make it fun for you: listen to music, enjoy the beautiful scenery, get a book on tape, enjoy your friends and neighbors, or just relish your time alone. You are going to feel great when you are done. Happy walking!

Chapter 6

You Really Are What You Eat!

Who's Really in Control?

Is it you or is it the food? Is it your head or is it your stomach? Is it you or is it your friends? How many times have you "thought with your stomach" and not with your head before you grabbed something to eat? How many times did you listen to your friends when they said "Come on, I know this is your favorite—just one isn't going to hurt you!" or "Come on, you're no fun." Well, it's no fun having diabetes or heart disease and they do hurt you.

How many times did you ignore your head when it was telling you to get up and exercise and the next thing you knew, you found yourself sitting on the couch eating bon-bons and watching *The Biggest Loser*? The people on that show didn't wake up one day two hundred pounds overweight. They got that way after years and years of not taking control. We all have the control; we just have to reclaim it.

For me, it took some time to train myself to understand that I am in control, that my brain controls what I do, not my stomach, not my taste buds, and certainly not another person. I still have days when I can't hear what my head is saying over the grumbling of my stomach and the screaming of my taste buds, but I refuse to surrender my control for too long. I definitely lose a few battles, but for now I am winning the war—and you can, too.

When I lose my battles, I will eat more than I should, but rarely—and I do mean rarely—do I put anything in my mouth that has harmful ingredients in it.

How many days does your body want to stay in bed in the morning but your brain says you have to go to work? Most of us listen to our brains at those moments because we really don't have a choice, we need to go to work to make our living. We get the oil changed in our cars because if we don't take care of the car, it will break down. We don't wait until the car is broken to take it to a mechanic; we have the oil changed and the tires rotated regularly. This is maintenance, and your body needs the same care and maintenance. Don't wait until your body is sick to take care of it.

Life is all about responsibility and control: responsibility to work, responsibility to take care of things we don't always want to address and most importantly, responsibility to take care of ourselves.

Control is not staying home all day and watching TV but going to work and being a productive member of society. Control is taking care of things that we view as a nuisance instead of giving in to a lackadaisical lifestyle. And control is saying no to things that are bad for your body and saying YES to health.

Start taking control today! No one else can eat better for you and no one else can exercise for you. Because it is something you do for yourself, when you reach your fitness goals, you have the greatest feelings because you can say with a clear conscience, I got here all by myself. I worked hard, I made sacrifices, I took control and I DID IT! Make the decision for health, you will see a new and improved you both physically and emotionally.

How to Curb Mindless Eating

How many times have you eaten something and had regrets afterward? How many times did you feel so full that you thought you could never eat again? And how often have you eaten something that was high in calories, cholesterol, or fat that you knew you should have avoided? We have all given in to this mindless overeating many times.

But that doesn't mean that we have to continue doing so.

Most of the eating we do is out of habit. We rarely eat because we are hungry or for the purpose of nutrition. But with persistence and awareness, we can break the habit of mindless eating.

If you find yourself eating mindlessly, look below and read the stages to becoming a mindful eater. It's all about awareness, control, and really taking the time to think about what we eat.

Stage 1 — *Mindless eating.* We eat whatever we want without giving it a thought. Then at some point we realize, This is not good, it's time for a change. This is the point where most of us start thinking about starting some diet as a quick fix. But diets are just short-term solutions.

Stage 2 — *Regret after we've indulged.* We go on eating whatever we want to eat, but now, after we eat it, we say to ourselves, Why did I just eat that? I shouldn't have eaten that. We feel guilty and we have regrets about it.

Stage 3 — *Regret while indulging.* We're still eating whatever we want, but at this step, as the food is in our mouth, we realize, I shouldn't be eating this—but keep on eating it anyway. After we eat it, we feel guilty and we have regrets.

Stage 4 — *Thinking before eating.* At this stage, we actually think about it before we eat it. We look at it, and say, I really shouldn't eat that, I don't really need that, and guess what—we eat in anyway! After we eat it, of course we feel guilty and we have regrets.

Stage 5 — *Still tempted, but successful.* At this stage, we think about it, we look at it and say, I really shouldn't eat that, I really don't need that, and guess what— I'm not going to eat it! SUCCESS! And then we feel proud and have absolutely no regrets.

Stage 6 — *Breaking the habit.* We are so well trained now that we don't even think about eating the forbidden foods. We just don't eat what we don't need. It's as natural as Stage 1 used to be.

For success, we need to retrain our minds, to change the way we think about food. Often we eat food to comfort us, to help us get through tough times. Although I have used food many times when I was upset, not once has it solved a single problem; it only makes me feel worse after I eat too much. I'm not saying that I don't reach for food today for the wrong reasons. Saying no is a lifelong struggle. I bounce back and forth between Stage 4 and Stage 6 often. If I am at Stage 6 and doing well for a while, as soon as I indulge myself more than once or twice in a short period of time, I have to start retraining myself, because I can easily start developing my bad habits again. Once you've been at Stage 6, it's much easier than it was the first time, but still takes some training and discipline. You need to make it a habit to talk to yourself before you grab for something so that you don't get caught up in the trap of mindless eating.

You have to ask yourself, What is stronger, my mind or my taste buds? I know—it's a close call for me, too. But you can strengthen your mind and win the battle of the bulge. We already know that strengthening your muscles helps with weight loss; so just remember this equation for success: strong mind + strong muscles = GREAT BODY!

Important Facts About Eating and Weight Loss

Changing the way you eat is such a challenge. If you are going to put the effort into changing your eating habits, here are some common mistakes you should avoid:

Not eating enough. Starving yourself is an ineffective and unhealthy way to lose weight. After approximately four hours of not eating, your metabolism will start to slow down. Be sure to eat something healthy every three to four hours.

Eliminating carbohydrates. Carbohydrates (carbs) are very important. Carbohydrates are the primary fuel source used by the body—do not take them out of your diet. Carbs are found in grains, fruits, vegetables, and dairy foods. You need carbs to burn fat. Fat metabolism depends on a continual breakdown of carbohydrates. A lot of the weight lost in the first weeks of a low-carb diet is water weight, not fat! In low-carbohydrates diets, muscle mass is lost, which may take pounds off the scale initially, but ultimately it will slow down your metabolism and you will gain the weight back, and then some.

Make sure you choose the right carbs. A Snickers bar is definitely not the best choice. Try a slice of whole wheat toast with a little bit of all natural peanut butter on it for a snack. You will be getting good carbs and some protein. Whole-grain cereals, brown rice, and fruits and vegetables are all great sources of carbohydrates.

Dieting without exercise. Dieting alone without exercise will result in the loss of lean mass. The best combination for weight loss is diet *and* exercise.

Losing too much weight too soon. The average body can only lose up to three pounds of fat per week, anything more than that is either water weight or muscle mass. Stay away from diets that promise a great amount of weight loss in a short time.

Judging your success based on the numbers on the scale. Muscle weighs three times more than fat. When you begin a diet and exercise routine it is possible that while you will most likely lose fat, you might see an increase in the number on the scale as your muscle mass increases and your body fat decreases. Use the way you feel in your clothing as your gauge, not the scale.

Diets, Diets, and More Diets

Do you have any idea how many diets there are out there? How many have you tried? Does anybody ever keep off the impressive amount of weight that can be lost on these diets? The truth is, some diets work temporarily, some diets don't work at all, and some diets aren't even safe.

Many diets are unrealistic, setting out too many restrictions that can't be maintained over the long term. The weight is usually put back on. It is said that 90 to 95 percent of people who lost weight, gained the weight back when they went off their diet.

My feeling is that if you have the willpower and discipline to go on one of these strict diets, you should definitely be able to make some permanent changes in your eating habits instead. The right changes can take the weight off and keep it off and will not deprive you; plus, you'll be healthier. The key is to make these changes permanent.

This is not very dramatic, but it could be time consuming at the beginning. You can continue to eat many of the foods you are used to eating (in moderation); you just may have to change the brand. There are some foods that are so bad that unfortunately changing brands won't cut it, so it is best to eliminate that food.

For starters, eat breakfast every day. A study by The National Weight Control Registry showed that 78 percent of people who lost more than thirty pounds and kept the weight off ate breakfast every day. People who skip breakfast tend to choose less nutritious foods and more convenient foods instead. Poor eating habits during the day leads to eating more throughout the day and into the evening.

Switch to whole grains. These are high in fiber, which makes you feel full, so you will eat less.

Drink six to eight glasses of water throughout the day. Drinking water before a meal can make you feel fuller. Dehydration slows down the fat-burning process. Also, now that you will be adding more whole grains to your diet, it is more important to drink enough water. Fiber does its best work in the digestive system when you are properly hydrated.

Don't eat before bed. Metabolism slows down in the evening hours. Try to stop eating at least two hours before bed. This is one of the harder ones for most people, but try to wean yourself off of those late-night snacks. Perhaps start by switching from cookies to an apple. Or stop eating 1 hour before bed for a while, and then stretch it to 1-½ hours etc.

Portion Control. What is a portion, anyway? Before you reach into that bag of pretzels, read the label and be sure to limit yourself to a portion.

Eat more fruits and vegetables. There are so many great ones. Fruits and veggies are good for you and are low in fat and calories.

No high fructose corn syrup (HFC). HFC is said to be one of the slowest metabolizing sugars and it is shown to cause cravings.

No artificial sweeteners. There have been many recent studies showing that artificial sweeteners actually make you want to eat more. These have also been shown to be potentially unhealthy; they should be eliminated from your diet. Look to natural, nutritious sweeteners such as honey, stevia, and molasses.

Hydrogenated oils (trans fats). Studies have shown that trans fatty acid consumption increases weight gain. Also, according to a study out of Harvard University, just one gram of trans fat is likely to increase the risk of heart disease by 20 percent, if consumed on a daily basis.

I think you will be surprised to find how many great healthy, low-fat and low-calorie foods are available. When I am eating my healthy foods I often say, "I love my new taste buds."

Regardless of the diets you've tried in the past, you can make real changes, be healthier, and lose weight. It is not as hard as you might think. The hardest part of this is getting used to reading labels, but regardless of your goals, you should know what is going into your body. You and only you should be in control of what you are eating, not Kraft, not General Mills, and definitely not the fast-food chains. A healthy, nutritious diet is the only proven way to lose weight and feel good—and it tastes good!

Who Says You Can't Eat Out and Eat Right?

If you are one of the many people who think you can't eat out and also eat right, fortunately, you are incorrect. I am happy to say that you can. Almost everything I eat at every meal is thought about. I seldom eat anything that I feel is not good for me. So, how then do I manage this when I go out? Let me put it this way, my husband's nickname for me is Substitute Sally.

When I go out, I never order directly off the menu. I always substitute something. Let's start with the salad; I don't let them put the dressing on my salad. Dressing is one of those things that I'm not willing to add extra calories to my waistline for. I will either eat my salad plain or put a little lemon juice on it. If I am eating Italian food, I will put tomato sauce on it (don't knock it till you've tried it). Next, if my dish comes with pasta on the side, I might opt for sautéed spinach instead. If I order coffee, half and half is out; I request skim milk or whatever milk they have that has fewer fat and calories than half and half. I keep stevia, a natural sweetener, with me and use that instead of sugar in my coffee. But usually I just stick with tea and lemon.

When I go out for breakfast I order a three-egg omelet made with one whole egg and two egg whites, with spinach and tomato inside, or onion. Whole-wheat toast holds the butter, and I substitute a tomato for the home fries. The waitress at the diner we go to knows most of my order before I even order!

Think of the calories saved with those substitutes—and I still get a great breakfast.

My sister-in-law teases me all the time about how I order, and jokes that it is embarrassing—she may even go to the ladies' room when I order. But recently, a group of us went out to dinner and as usual I substituted several items. At the end of the meal, the owner came over and asked us who had ordered the special meal. My sister-in-law said it was me: "We try not to take her anywhere because she substitutes everything whenever she goes out." He said, "No, not all. I thought the substitution was great. It was a nice combination. So much so that we are adding it to the menu as we speak."

So don't feel uncomfortable, order what you like. Even though my sister-in-law jokes with me, she really respects what I do, as do the rest of my friends and family. As for the restaurants, if you go to a restaurant that can't honor a few fairly simple requests, you might want to find a new place to dine. After all, you are the customer and it is their job to make sure your meal is to your liking. Besides, you never know—maybe the owner will add your special order to the menu. Bon appétit.

Can You Have Your Cake and Eat It, Too?

Let's take a look at a regular box of cake mix with frosting, the kind we use to make our kids' birthday cakes with, and the mix and frosting that are used to make the cupcakes that are frequently eaten in school, at our children's parties, and sold at the bake sales.

When ingredients are listed on a label, they begin with the highest amount of an ingredient in the product and go to the lowest amount. So there is more of the first ingredient than the ingredients that follow. This is from a regular boxed cake mix:

The first ingredient is sugar.

The second ingredient in the mix is enriched bleached flour. Bleached flour is just that, flour that is bleached.

The third ingredient is partially hydrogenated soybean oil. Hydrogenated oils cause obesity and can cause diarrhea and malnutrition. The USDA's dietary guidelines recommend keeping trans fatty acid consumption as low as possible. Partially hydrogenated oils or trans fatty acids increase total cholesterol levels and LDL levels (bad cholesterol), and reduce HDL levels (good cholesterol). Simply put, trans fatty acids are very bad for your heart.

The next ingredient is propylene glycol. According to the safety data sheets of industrial chemical manufacturers available at safteylab.com, chemicals such as this one cause damage to the central nervous system. Propylene glycol is a clear liquid used in antifreeze and de-icing solutions.

Next, we have sodium aluminum phosphate. There is a strong connection between aluminum and Alzheimer's disease.

As I go down the label of the cake mix a little further, I come to more hydrogenated oils.

The final ingredient is artificial flavors. I don't know about you, but I prefer my flavors to be natural, not a substance that was processed in a lab to mimic the real thing.

Then there's the frosting:

The first two ingredients are powdered sugar and sugar.

Next comes more partially hydrogenated oil.

So can you have your cake and eat it, too?

From time to time, you can. Keep in mind that a piece of cake is a treat. The Dr. Oetker brand makes a cake mix which contains about eight ingredients, all of which are organic. Arrowhead Mills also makes an organic cake mix. For frosting, I have switched to homemade whipped cream—yes, it is fattening, but far less dangerous than the traditional frostings available in the supermarket. I mix heavy cream and honey with a hand mixer. Be sure to use it sparingly.

A treat should be something that makes you happy, not sick somewhere down the road. And of course, moderation is the key. I am not suggesting that we indulge daily in cake, organic or otherwise, but when you do decide to have a piece, let it be something healthful, not toxic. An organic-ingredients cake with homemade frosting is delicious.

Although the sugar content is slightly lower in the organic cake mix, it is still high in sugar and should probably be avoided if you are a diabetic. Read the labels of the food you eat. Then decide whether or not it's good enough for your precious body.

Know what you are putting in your body and then make the choice. If you are concerned about the price, the organic cake mix is about $1.20 more than the other brands regular price. I'd say that's a small price to pay to help preserve your health.

Do We Really All Scream for Ice Cream?

I hope not! But if you do, I'd like to offer you a healthy ice cream but the word "cream" in ice cream makes it hard to come up with a healthy alternative. But I do have some good alternatives for you.

Stonyfield's nonfat Gotta Have Vanilla frozen yogurt has just 100 calories in half a cup, no fat, and only seven ingredients. You also get the advantage of the yogurt cultures without a lot of calories.

If yogurt won't cut it and you must have ice cream, here are some suggestions:

Haagen-Dazs has a line called Five. It is called Five because it only has five ingredients. When it comes to ingredients, less is best! Some of the ice creams have a really long list of ingredients, which consist of many words I can't even pronounce. Five has 220 calories in half a cup, better than what you could be eating but still a lot of calories.

Haagen-Dazs regular vanilla bean ice cream has only a few more ingredients, and also a few more calories. The regular vanilla has 290 calories per half cup, and lets face it, who's eating just half a cup? That means that eating a cup would mean consuming 140 less calories in the Haagen-Dazs Five. I can definitely do without the extra 140 calories.

Horizon organic ice cream has 170 calories per half a cup with seven ingredients and is all organic.

Breyers All Natural now has a new ice cream called Smooth and Dreamy, also only seven ingredients and only 110 calories per half a cup.

Purely Decadent ice cream is made with agave nectar instead of sugar, and coconut milk. It's dairy-free and sugar-free, yet still all natural. It has eight organic ingredients with 150 calories in half a cup. This is my favorite because it has no refined sugar.

One year I was at my son's end-of-the-year ice cream party. One of the moms brought in the Breyers All Natural ice cream and another mom brought in another brand, the name of which I don't recall. It was a very hot day, and by the end of the party, the Breyers ice cream had melted, it was more like a shake than ice cream. The other brand wasn't melted at all. It had so many preservatives in it that it didn't even melt.

YUK!

I generally try to stay away from ice cream—it doesn't look nearly as good on my hips as it does in the bowl. I bought an ice-cream maker for those times that I'd like to indulge in a little ice-cream. I use Bolthouse chocolate milk and just throw it in and in half an hour it's done. It is more like a soft-serve ice cream. It has 150 calories in a cup and no added sugar.

Sometimes, instead of ice cream, I make myself shakes because I can make them healthy. I love the pina colada shake, which is half a can of natural coconut milk, one can of pineapple in its own juice, and a banana to thicken it; and ice. You can add any fruits and mix with apple juice or milk and enjoy a refreshing, healthy, low-calorie snack.

If you must indulge and have ice cream, just make sure it melts on a hot day and do it in moderation.

Sugar: How Sweet It Isn't

How can something that tastes so good be so bad for you? Although sugar comes from a plant, by the time it gets to us, it is so heavily processed that it can hardly be called natural any longer.

When my daughter was twelve years old, she was always tired and constantly complained of aches and pains. She would come home from school and just lie down on the couch. Her doctor kept her out of gym because she was in too much pain to play. She went for many different tests. We tried massage therapy, physical therapy, and she got adjusted at the chiropractor. I had her braces taken off in case something in the braces was bothering her. Nothing helped.

Finally my chiropractor began nutrition response testing in his practice. Nutritonal response testing is a way of analyzing the body to determine causes of illness. He tested her for various things and it turned out that she had sensitivity to refined sugars. We eliminated these sugars from her diet, and the transformation was unbelievable. Within a couple of weeks, she was back in gym, running track, and dancing. My daughter could not sit still. She now had the energy that a twelve-year-old should have, and then some!

Maybe you don't have the symptoms my daughter had, but that's not to say that sugar is not hurting you in ways you don't know about. Sugar, which is highly addictive, is one of the major contributors to obesity in this country. Sugar increases the risk of diabetes, and can even lead to depression.

Sugar weakens the immune system, which leaves one more susceptible to illnesses. It is known to contribute to arthritis and can cause headache. We all know sugar leads to tooth decay, but it can also exacerbate PMS symptoms and cause fatigue. In addition, there has been a lot of information linking sugar to cancer. That's enough for me to stay away from it.

There is a lot of evidence about how sugar is bad for the body, but not one proven benefit of refined sugar. Refined sugars contain no nutritional value; they are filled with empty calories.

To satisfy your cravings for sweets, try adding more natural sugars to your diet. Some alternatives are honey, stevia, maple syrup, and xylitol. Fruits and vegetables are a great source of natural sugars.

I know it's nearly impossible to eliminate refined sugars altogether, but try to keep them to a minimum. Read your labels and know how much sugar is in your food. Then make the decision to eat it or leave it. I try to keep my foods under five grams of refined sugar per serving.

Are You Reading Your Labels?

In order to eat healthy, you need to know what is going into your body. The first part of the label that I look at is the ingredients label. If there are ingredients in the food that I'm not willing to put into my body, then there is no reason to look at the label any further. I don't want artificial this or artificial that in my food. No high fructose corn syrup, nothing bleached, and no hydrogenated oils are going into my body if I can help it. It is important to remember that hydrogenated oils are trans fats. The nutritional values list on the label may say that there are no trans fats, but in fact if it has .5 grams or less, it is acceptable, for some reason, to declare that the product has zero trans fats. To me, zero should mean zero! Read the ingredients and avoid foods that list hydrogenated and partially hydrogenated oils of any kind.

When you read the ingredients on the label, the ingredients with the greatest amount go first and the ingredients with the least amount go last. Stay away from foods that have sugar listed as one of the 1ˢᵗ few ingredients. Try to keep sugar toward the end of that list. Always check the nutritional values, then determine how much is considered a serving. Sometime we may eat an item and see that it is 100 calories and think that's great. But if that is 100 calories per serving, and there are three servings in the item, it becomes 300 calories. And with snack or treat items, it is so easy to eat more than one serving without even thinking about it. Calories come from carbohydrates, protein and fat.

Next you want to look at fats. Trans fats should be avoided altogether. Saturated fats are also best to avoid because they increase the risk of heart disease. Polyunsaturated and monounsaturated fats keep your heart healthy. These are good fats.

Cholesterol can also contribute to heart disease, keep it low.

Sodium can be found in the most surprising foods—and in large amounts. I am often amazed to see how much sodium is in foods you wouldn't even expect to contain sodium. Pay close attention to this. Some canned soups can have close to 1,000 mg of sodium per serving. Sodium should be kept below 2400 mg, so be very careful. If the can of soup is two servings and you eat the whole can, you could be eating as much as 2,000 mg of sodium in just your lunch. Some sodium is necessary for our hearts and kidneys, but be aware of how much you're consuming, the numbers add up fast.

Carbohydrates are sugar, fiber, and other starches. Carbohydrates are a source of energy. There are good carbs and bad carbs. Bad carbs are carbohydrates that are refined to remove much of its nutritional value. Good Carbs are high in fiber and nutrients so do not eliminate these from your diet.

Fiber is one you can keep high. Most Americans don't consume enough fiber. If you're eating the right foods, it's not too difficult to get the recommend daily values of fiber. Fiber also keeps us full longer. Strive for 20–35 grams of fiber daily, depending on your age and gender. Men need more fiber then women and after the age of 50 the recommended amounts decrease.

Sugars can come from natural sources such as fruit, vegetables, and dairy products, or they can be added sugars. This part of the label does not specify the source of the sugar; go to the list of ingredients to determine where the sugars are coming from.

Protein is important for the growth and repair of muscles, blood, and organs.

Percentage of Daily Values: Try to keep these numbers at 100 percent daily from a variety of different foods.

Make sure you know what you are eating because knowledge is power—the power to eat and live healthier. Health is a big contributor to happiness and well-being. We get one chance on this earth, so make it a happy and healthy experience. An unhealthy diet does not lead to a happier life, but a healthy diet can lead to a happier life.

What's On Your Mind?

What follows is a question from a reader/client of mine. I've been asked a lot of questions about these topics, so I thought I would share them with you.

Dear Robin,

One of my New Year's resolutions is to eat healthier. I don't want to think of it as a diet but as a lifestyle change. My question for you is, What is best, low fat or fat free; whole wheat or multigrain; "good carbs" or no carbs; three meals a day or five small ones; eight 8-ounce glasses of water or more; jump on the scale daily, weekly, or not at all? And then there are people who say eat nothing white. Can you shed some light on these conflicting views?

Thanks in advance,

Mary Elizabeth – Blue Point

Congratulations to you on making the choice to eat healthier, I know it sounds a little clichéd, but you really are what you eat.

Low fat is better than fat free. Quite often, in fat-free foods, sugars have been added to compensate for the lack of fat. They often have the same amount of calories as the regular version and in some instances may have even more calories. In addition, many fat-free foods add HVP (hydrolyzed vegetable proteins), another name for MSG, or monosodium glutamate, which should be avoided. It is just substituting one bad thing for another. Stay away from all trans fats, and keep saturated fats to a minimum. Some fats are necessary, so keep it low-fat.

Whole wheat and multigrain are both great choices. Just make sure it is 100 percent whole wheat. Carbs are a very important part of your diet. It can be quite confusing because there are good carbs and bad carbs. But definitely do not give them up. Make sure they come from whole grains; you should avoid white flours as much as possible; it is quite difficult to eliminate white flour completely from your diet, but definitely keep it to a minimum.

Breads that are not made from whole wheat or whole grain flour lack many of the vitamins and minerals, and much of the fiber, found in breads made from whole-grain flours. Milling and processing results in … white bread! And when the vitamins and minerals are removed, your body absorbs the nutrients differently. The body breaks down enriched flour too fast, and too much sugar enters the bloodstream at one time. This causes quick highs and lows in your blood-sugar level, which can cause mood swings and tiredness and can lead to Type 2 diabetes and obesity. With refined flour, you're not getting close to the amount of nutrients that you'd benefit from with whole grains. In addition, the flour is often bleached to make it white, and that is as bad as it sounds.

Water is extremely important, however we do get water from many sources other than drinking it from a glass. If you eat lots of fruits and vegetables, you are getting water from that source as well. The exact amount of water needed is different for everyone based on diet, physical activity, and body size. My suggestion would be to make water your beverage of choice. Water is extremely important to overall health and it can help keep your eating under control. It is said that our bodies can confuse thirst for hunger, so strive for eight 8-ounce glasses daily.

Five small meals a day is definitely the way to go. It keeps your metabolism working all day. After about three to four hours without eating, your metabolism slows down. It is not a good idea at all to let yourself become hungry. If you eat five small meals, you are more likely to make wiser eating choices as well because you are not being driven by hunger.

Once we become hungry we grab what's quick and easy, and although an apple or banana is quick and easy, for some reason, when we're hungry, the cookies and candy usually win. A handful of nuts between meals are a great snack.

As far as getting on the scale, I think that's a personal preference. Personally, I keep my time on the scale to a minimum. I find that if I get on the scale when I've gained weight, I get upset—and what do most of us do when we get upset? We grab something to eat. If I get on the scale and I've lost weight, I congratulate myself and then I grab something to eat. So for me, the scale doesn't work so well. I use my clothing as my gauge. Your clothing doesn't lie. When you get dressed in the morning, do you feel good, or do your clothes feel tight and uncomfortable?

There are studies that suggest that people who weigh themselves regularly are more successful at maintaining a healthy weight because they catch themselves as soon as they start to put on any weight. So—there is no wrong or right here. Just do what works for you.

I commend you for making an effort to eat well in order to enjoy optimum health; and it is best to combine a healthy diet with exercise. The combination is a great duo. You will look great and feel great. And you are correct in calling it a lifestyle change. Approximately 90 percent of those who go on a diet gain the weight back at some point. If you look around, will probably see that this is an accurate statistic. You can't diet forever, but hopefully, you can change your eating habits forever with the occasional slip-up, which is okay.

You Really Are What You Eat!

Rockin' Robin Menu

*Breakfast Suggestions *

Bowl of Cheerios with Banana

Arrowhead Mills Kamut Flakes

Homemade Oatmeal with Walnuts, Raisins &
Cinnamon and a Dash of Nutmeg

2 Eggs with Whole-Wheat Toast

Matthews's Whole-Wheat English Muffins with
Natural Peanut Butter Or Polaner All-Fruit

Nature's Path Waffles or Van's Flax Waffles with
Fresh or Frozen Fruit on Top

Nature's Path Agave Granola Cereal with Chobani
Plain or Honey Yogurt

Whole-Wheat French Toast
Healthy Muffins (see recipe in chapter 8)
Pumpkin Pancakes (see chapter 8)

*Lunch Suggestions *

Organic Bean Burrito (Costco) with Broccoli
Sprouts & Avocado

Veggie Wrap (Nature's Promise Whole-Wheat Wrap
or Traders Whole-Wheat Wrap) Put Your
Favorite Veggies in It. Change it Up for Variety

All Natural Peanut Butter With Polaner All-Fruit on
One of the Following Breads: Nature's
Promise Breads Or Pepperidge Farm Naturals
Bread, Whole-Wheat Or Multigrain
Nature's Pride Whole-Wheat Bread, Matthews
Whole-Wheat Bread, or Kirkland Organic Whole-
Wheat Bread

All Natural Soups with a Slice of
Natural Whole-Wheat Bread

(Trader Joe's Has Lots of Soups that
Don't Contain MSG)

Boar's Head Turkey on Whole-Wheat Wrap
or Bread with Lettuce, Tomato and Honey
Mustard or a Small Amount of Mayo

Tuna Salad or Chicken Salad with Balsamic Vinegar

You Really Are What You Eat!

Dinner Suggestions

(Add Vegetable of Your Choice)

Turkey Meatball Hero with Whole-Wheat Bread

Turkey Hotdog

Spinach Whole-Wheat Veggie Pizza
(Hold the Cheese — You Won't Even Miss the
Cheese with All the Veggies)

Whole-Wheat Pasta with Spinach and Sauce or Add
Your Favorite Veggies

Organic Chicken with Veggies Sautéed in Olive Oil
with Brown Rice

Macaroni with Beans (Sauté Garlic in Olive Oil) And
Heinz Vegetarian Baked Beans, Add to
the Small Pasta Shells

Salad: Romaine Lettuce, Cucumber, Broccoli
Sprouts, Tomato, Black Beans, Avocado, and Corn
with Chicken Strips (Put Leftover Salad in a Wrap
for Tomorrow's Lunch)

Rockin' Robin's Handbook to a Healthier Life

All Natural Lentil Soup over Whole-Wheat Pasta

Grilled Wild Alaskan Salmon (Not Farm Raised)

Harvestland Organic Chicken

Madras Lentils over Whole-Wheat Pasta

You Really Are What You Eat!

Snack Suggestions

Apples or Bananas with All Natural Peanut Butter

All Fresh Fruits and Veggies

Handful of Nuts

Stonyfield or Chobani Yogurt (Plain; Add Your Own
Fruit and Cinnamon or Cocoa Powder)

1 oz of Dark Chocolate

Trader Joe's Blue Bag of Popcorn

Sweet Potato (Baked)

Plain Rice Cakes with Peanut Butter

Triscuts

Bolthouse

Lara Bars

*Beverage Suggestions *

Water, Water, Water!

Green Tea

Homemade Iced Tea Made with Honey

Water with Orange Slices or Lemon Wedges

Fat-Free Milk
100% Fruit Juices

*Nature's Promise is Stop & Shop's All Natural Line

Chapter 7

Holiday Season Strategies

Tips for Keeping Off those Extra Holiday Pounds

Tis the season when we all tend to put on a few extra pounds. This year let's try to break that cycle and say *no* to putting on extra pounds. It can be done.

Say no. First, we have to break the habit of saying *yes* to everything and get into the habit of saying *no* to ourselves. Just because it's the holiday season is no excuse to sacrifice our health and our waistline. Holiday time does not mean there are no limits. Set boundaries this year and try your hardest to stick to them.

Say yes. Although boundaries are important, you are entitled to indulge sometimes but don't over-indulge.

Eat. Eat an apple, a pear, or a cup of cereal before you go to a party. If you go to a party hungry, all reasoning will go out the window and you will just start eating everything. If you're not hungry when you arrive, you will tend to make wiser choices and not over-indulge.

Have a plan, Before you go to the holiday party, have a plan. Decide what you will indulge in and what you will say no to. Remember, you can't say yes to everything and escape the holiday with your waistline intact. It's a choice. Your body or the cake?

Bring a healthy alternative. Whenever I go to a party, I bring either a fruit salad or a vegetable platter so I know I won't be tempted to eat the chips or the cake.

Beware of all those office snacks! I don't work in an office, but my clients tell me all about those tempting snacks that are offered almost daily. Just because it's there doesn't mean you have to eat it. Pick one day a week that will be your day to indulge, not over-indulge, on office snacks.

Exercise. Don't neglect your exercise program. Yes, we are all very busy at this time of the year, but your body is still a priority. No matter how hard we try, we will all be taking in a few extra calories, but maybe that can be offset by exercising. You couldn't put anything else on hold for six weeks and expect it to stay the way you left it—the same holds true for your body and your health.

Make choices. Next time you're at a party, make a choice, chips or dessert. It's all about setting boundaries. You really don't need both. And remember, you can always bring something, a gesture that's always appreciated.

Do the math. Next time you're about to indulge, try to calculate the calories you are about to consume. It might just make you rethink the cake.

Believe in yourself. Tell yourself that you can say no, that snacks and cakes are not more important than your health. Think about how lousy you will feel if you can't button your pants after the holidays are long gone. Let's make this the year with no "gifts" of extra holiday pounds.

I wish you a happy and healthy holiday season spent with good friends, family, and healthy foods. It's up to you to make it a healthier one.

Post-Holiday Tips

The holiday season should be a healthy and joyful time of the year. But often during the holiday season we lose sight of how much we are really eating. Those extra calories not only contribute to weight gain, they also may contribute to some health problems. Research has shown that most of us gain about one pound during the holidays. That doesn't sound too bad, but after ten years, that's an easy ten pounds. The next problem is many of us continue eating too much after the holiday season, pushing that one pound to two pounds, three pounds, or even more. Those who are already overweight are more likely to gain at least five pounds during this time.

Not only is the weight gain often uncomfortable, significant weight gain is a contributor to heart disease, high blood pressure, diabetes, and certain cancers. Here are some tips to getting your pre-holiday waistline back.

Start today. Not later—today! Don't put off until tomorrow what you can do today.

Set realistic goals. Don't strive for perfection, that's not happening for any of us. Just strive to be the best YOU.

Get rid of the junk. Fill your pantry with foods that will support better eating. Get rid of the cookies and candy. I don't mean get rid of it by eating it, either!

Keep a food journal. You'll be surprised how much picking we all do during the day. You may think twice about eating something if you have to stop and write it down. A food journal is a great way to kick-start a diet.

Exercise. Jump on that treadmill. I'm sure some of you are saying, I don't have the time. A wise man once told me that when you say you don't have the time for something, what you really mean is that it's not really important enough to you. I'm often amazed by the hectic lives that some of my clients have. They have jobs, kids, school, and families and yet they are committed to their workouts. This is because it's important enough to them to make the time for it. How important is it to you?

Join a gym. Studies show that those who exercised at a gym are more likely to stick with their routine.

Make fitness a priority. Eventually it will just become a way of life for you. Exercise will make you feel great; you will start looking forward to your next workout. I've seen it happen over and over again. Many of my clients start off exercising because they need to and continue doing it because they want to. Give it a whirl; you might just surprise yourself.

What's Your New Year's Resolution?

Many people resolve to lose weight, quit smoking, or start a fitness program on New Year's Eve. I don't usually make New Year's resolutions. Although it is great to make a resolution to change things in your life, why wait until January 1st? If you want to change your job or change your hairstyle, do you wait for the new year to make that change? Probably not! So why wait when it comes to quality of life or health issues?

As you may remember, I said earlier that for part of my life I was a junk-food eater. My face would light up if I saw a Twix bar, and I'd think nothing of having cookies for breakfast if I so desired. In April of 2005, at thirty-eight, I decided that it was time I started eating healthier. I called it my New Life resolution. I didn't do it because the calendar changed, I did it for me. I've stuck to my resolution for over five years (with a little cheat now and again). Not only am I proud of my accomplishment, but also my body is so much better for it. I benefited from my resolution both emotionally and physically.

So if it happens to be New Year's Eve, go ahead and make that resolution to quit smoking, eat healthier, or start a fitness program. Just make it your New Life resolution, not a New Year's resolution. That way, after all the hoopla of the new year has come and gone, your resolution will still be a part of your New Life.

I wish you strength, determination, and success in whatever New Life resolution you choose. And I wish you and your family a happy and healthy new year.

Happy New Year and Happy New You!

I can't believe it's 2010. Where does the time go? Time goes so fast that we need to cherish every day. I hope 2010 is a happy year for all of you. Regardless of what's going on in our lives, it's very difficult to be happy and enjoy each day to the fullest if you're not healthy.

So for the new year, why not focus on a new you? A new and improved healthier you, which means a new and improved *happier* you.

Most of us have some habit we can kick that will improve our health. Maybe it's too many sweets, or maybe it's smoking, or eating fried fatty foods? Maybe instead of kicking a habit, we have to make a new improved habit. It could be eating more fruits and veggies or it could be starting an exercise pro-gram—or even learning to relax. Maybe you need to get more sleep at night or maybe you can work on not sweating the small stuff in life.

Any and all of these can lead to a new and improved you, and what better way to start the new year then with a healthier you!

Take control where you can. We don't ever have 100 percent control, but we do have some control. Take advantage of it, and don't be a victim of your own bad habits or your lack of good ones. You owe it to yourself and you owe it to those who love you to take the best possible care of your body and mind that you can.

Chapter 8

Rockin' Robin Recipes

Muffins

Banana Muffins _makes 12 muffins; aprox. 135 calories each_

Preheat oven to 325

3 Large Ripe Bananas

1/3 Cup Honey

1 tbsp. Stevia Powder

1 Egg White

4 tbsp. Applesauce

1–1/2 Cups Whole-Wheat Flour

1 tsp. Baking Soda

Pinch of Salt

Mix all ingredients and pour into greased muffin pans, bake 14–17 minutes or until toothpick comes out clean.

Blueberry Whole Wheat Muffins _makes 12 muffins; aprox. 130 calories each_

Preheat oven to 400

2/3 Cup Oat Bran

1–1/3 Cups Whole-Wheat flour

1/4 Cup Honey

1/2 tbsp. Stevia Powder

3–1/2 tsp. Baking Powder

1/2 tsp. Baking Soda

2 tbsp. Cinnamon

1/2 tsp. Nutmeg (optional)

1 Egg

8 oz. + 1tbsp. Unsweetened Applesauce

1/2 Cup Skim Milk

1 tsp. Vanilla Extract

1 Cup Blueberries (or Your Favorite Berries)

Sprinkle of Ground Flaxseeds (optional)

Nuts (Optional)

Spray 12-cup muffin tin with cooking spray. Mix all ingredients together. Pour into tins. Bake 15–17 minutes or until toothpick comes out clean.

Chocolate Zucchini Muffins   *makes 12 muffins; aprox. 82 calories each*

Preheat oven to 350 degrees

1 Cup Whole-Wheat Flour	1/3 Cup Honey
1/3 Cup Cocoa Powder	3/4 tbsp. Stevia Powder
1/4 tsp. Cinnamon	1 tsp. Baking Soda

1/2 Cup Skim Milk	1/4 Cup Unsweetened Applesauce
2 tsp. Vinegar	1 Egg, Beaten
1 tsp. Vanilla	

1/3 Cup Grated Zucchini	1/2 Cup Boiling Water

Mix flour, honey, stevia, cocoa, cinnamon, and baking soda in one bowl. In another bowl, mix milk, vinegar, applesauce, egg, and vanilla. Pour into cocoa mixture and mix by hand. Add zucchini, then the boiling water. (The mixture will be thin.)

Bake 17–20 minutes or until toothpick comes out clean.

Enjoy!

Zucchini Carrot Muffins   *makes 24 muffins; aprox. 80 calories each*

Preheat oven to 400 degrees

2 Cups Whole-Wheat Flour

2 Cups Unsweetened Applesauce

1 Cup Oat Flour or Oatmeal

2 tsp. Vanilla Extract

1 tsp. Baking Soda

1/2 tbsp. Stevia Powder and 1/2 Cup Honey

1 tsp. Baking Powder

1 Cup Shredded Carrots*

1 tbsp. Ground Cinnamon

1 Cup Shredded Zucchini*

2 Egg Whites, 1 Whole Egg

Lightly grease 24 muffin cups. In a bowl, sift together the flour, baking soda, baking powder, and cinnamon. In another bowl, beat together eggs, applesauce, honey, stevia,and vanilla. Mix the flour mixture into the egg mixture. Fold in the carrots and zucchini and banana.

Bake 18 to 20 minutes or until a toothpick comes out clean. Let cool completely.

*Mixed berries may be substituted for the carrots and zucchini.

<u>Whole Grain Fruit & Cream Muffins</u> *makes 12 muffins; aprox. 145 calories each*

Preheat oven to 350 degrees

1–1/4 Cups Whole-Wheat Flour

1/2 Cup Quick Oats

1/3 Cup Honey + 1/2 tbsp. Stevia Powder

1/3 Cup Oat Bran

2–1/2 tsp. Baking Powder

1 tbsp. Cinnamon

1 Cup Fresh Or Frozen Fruit

1 Cup Skim Milk

3 tbsp. Applesauce

2 tsp. Vanilla Extract

1 Egg

Sprinkle of Ground Flaxseed

Cream Filling

1/2 Cup Low-Fat Cream Cheese

1 tbsp. Honey

1/4 Cup Berries or Diced Peaches

Spray 12 muffin-tin cups with non-stick spray. Combine dry ingredients in a medium bowl and mix well. Add milk, applesauce, vanilla, and egg to dry ingredients. Stir fruit in another bowl with cream cheese and honey. Blend and add 1/4 cup of the fruit. Spoon half of the mixture equally into muffin tins. Place 1 teaspoon of cream cheese mixture in center of each, then cover with remaining batter.

Bake 20 to 25 minutes or until toothpick comes out clean.

Makes 12–14 muffins.

Breakfast

<u>Whole-Wheat Pancakes</u> *makes 8 pancakes, 168 calories each*

1–2/3 Cups Whole-Wheat Flour	1 tsp. Pure Vanilla Extract
1/3 Cup Oats or Wheat Germ	1 Cup Unsweetened Applesauce
1/2 tsp. Baking Soda	1/4 Cup Plain Yogurt
1–1/2 tsp. Baking Powder	1 Cup Skim Milk
1/2 tbsp. Stevia Powder	2 Eggs, Beaten
2 tbsp. Honey	2 tbsp. Cinnamon

In a large bowl combine all ingredients and mix well. Heat a frying pan over medium heat and grease with cooking spray. Pour in mixture. When bubbles form on top of the pancake, flip it over and cook on other side for about 2–3 minutes.

Pumpkin Pancake Recipe   *makes 7 pancakes, aprox. 235 calorie each*

1/2 Cup Whole-Wheat Flour

1/2 Cup Oat Bran

3 tbsp. Honey

1 tsp. Baking Powder

1/2 tsp. Baking Soda

Pinch of Salt

1–1/2 tbsp. Cinnamon

1/4 tsp. Nutmeg

1 Egg

1 Cup Plain Low Fat Yogurt Or Plain Applesauce

1/2 Can of Pumpkin

Mix all ingredients, spray pan with cooking spray, and cook over medium heat until top bubbles and edges are slightly dry; flip over and cook 2–3 minutes.

Stuffed French Toast

Preheat oven to 350 degrees

1 Loaf of Whole-Wheat Bread, Cut into Cubes

6 Whole Eggs

4 Egg Whites

1/2 Cup Organic Fat-Free Milk

1/2 Cup Pure Maple Syrup

1 tsp. Pure Vanilla Extract

1 tbsp. Cinnamon

1/4 tsp. Nutmeg (optional)

Frozen Mixed Berries (or Banana)

Mix milk, eggs, vanilla, and maple syrup in a bowl and set aside. Spray a 13" x 9" baking pan with cooking spray. Put a layer of cubed bread on the bottom. Pour half the egg mixture over the bread and cover with mixed berries. Add the rest of the cubed bread. Cover with remaining egg mixture. Soak overnight. Bake, covered, for 25 minutes and bake uncovered for another 10-15 minutes or until cooked thoroughly.

Vegetables

Spinach Balls   _Makes 30 Spinach Balls, approx. 16 calories each_

1 Bag of Frozen Spinach (thawed and drained)

1 Egg

1/2 Cup Flavored Breadcrumbs

1/4 Cup Grated Cheese

Coat a baking sheet with olive oil. Roll into balls and bake at 350 until light brown, about 15 minutes.

Spinach and Pasta

1 Pound Whole-Wheat, Multigrain, Or Brown Rice Pasta

1 Can of Whole Tomatoes (chopped)

1 Bag Of Fresh Spinach or Frozen Spinach (thawed and drained)

2–3 Garlic Cloves

Grated Cheese

Sauté garlic in olive oil, add spinach and cook until soft. Add chopped tomatoes. Cook until heated and pour over pasta. Add grated cheese to taste.

Veggie Frittata

3 Cups of Your Favorite Veggies

4 Whole Eggs

3 Egg Whites

Sauté the veggies in about 2 tablespoons f olive oil over medium heat until soft. In a bowl, mix eggs with a little water, salt and pepper. Pour veggies into greased baking pan, cover with egg mixture. Bake at 350 until egg mixture is cooked.

*Tip: Sauté extra veggies and pour over whole-wheat pasta for tomorrow's dinner; if desired, add tomato sauce.

Beverages

Healthy Non-Alcoholic Pina Colada

1 Can Pineapple in Pineapple Juice

1/2 Can All Natural Coconut Milk

Crushed Ice

Banana To Thicken (optional)

Mix all ingredients in a blender until smooth.

Fruit Shake

1 Cup Fat-Free Milk

1/3 Cup Frozen Fruit of Your Choice

Crushed Ice (optional)

Mix in blender and enjoy!

Iced Tea

8 Tea Bags, Any Flavor

1/2 Gallon Boiling Water

1/4 to 1/2 Cup Honey

1 tbsp. Stevia Powder

Steep tea bags, honey, and stevia in boiling water for about half an hour. Add ice.

Healthy Hot Chocolate

1 Cup Organic Skim Milk

2–1/2 tsp. Dark Chocolate Cocoa Powder

2 tbsp. Honey

Pour milk into a pot over medium heat, stir in cocoa powder and honey until blended and hot.

Desserts

<u>**Ginger Cookies**</u> *makes 36 cookies; approx. 96 calories each*

Preheat oven to 350

3/4 Cup Grape Seed Oil	1 Cup Honey
1 tsp. Baking Soda	2 tsp. Ginger
1 tbsp. Cinnamon	1 Egg
2–1/4 Cups Whole-Wheat Flour	1/2 Cup Raisins (optional)

Mix together with electric mixer, shape into 1–1/2" balls, and bake for 12-15 minutes. Enjoy!

<u>Chocolate Tofu Cheesecake</u> *makes 8 servings, approx. 190 calories each without berries*

Preheat oven to 350

Crust:

1–1/2 Cups Chocolate Cookie Crumbs (Annie's Chocolate Bunnies, crushed)

1 tbsp. Vanilla Extract

2 tbsp. Grape Seed Oil

Cheesecake:

8 oz. Tofu

1/2 Cup Part-Skim Ricotta Cheese

4 oz. Light Cream Cheese (for a slightly lower calorie version, substitute 4 oz. Chobani Plain Yogurt)

1/3 Cup Pure Maple Syrup

2 Egg Whites

1 Egg

3 tbsp. Vanilla Extract

1/4 Cup Dark Chocolate Cocoa Powder

Mix the cookie crumbs with the oil and vanilla and press into a 9" spring-form pan. In a food processor or blender, combine remaining ingredients and puree until smooth. Spread over the crust and bake for 1 hour. Chill in the refrigerator overnight before serving. Add raspberries on top, if desired.

Chapter 9

Keeping Your Healthy Foods Healthy

How Are You Cooking All this Healthy Food?

I hope that you have made the decision to start eating to nurture your body and fuel it up for all that is expected of it. But now we have to make sure you are preparing it in a safe manner.

I know the microwave is such a convenient way of heating and cooking food, but how much are you willing to gamble for that convenience?

Research conducted by Doctors Hertel and Blanc has confirmed that microwaving food decreases its nutritional value. Studies also show that people who ate microwaved food had a decrease in HDL ("good" cholesterol) and a decrease in white blood cells, which kill germs. The radiation is thought to affect the central nervous system, possibly causing headaches, backaches, and disorientation. Microwaving food in plastic wrap is carcinogenic. If you must microwave your food, cover it with a paper towel instead of plastic wrap.

An alternative to the microwave is a convection oven. It is not as fast as a microwave oven, but it is faster than your traditional oven. A convection oven cooks in one-third the time of a traditional oven. It is simply an oven that uses a fan to expedite the cooking time. I have a toaster/convection oven and it is great.

What about your pots and pans? What are they made out of? If you are using non-stick pans, you probably are not going to be happy to hear this, but I am telling you because I care. Non-stick pans, at high temperatures, emit toxic gases, which are linked to hundreds, perhaps thousands, of pet bird deaths and an unknown number of human illnesses each year, according to tests commissioned by the Environmental Working Group (EWG).

The good news is that there is an alternative. Cuisinart has a line of cookware called Greenware. These feature a ceramic-based surface—perfect for cooking, and non-stick, too.

If you're going to invest your time and effort in cooking and eating healthy food, keep it healthy from start to finish. Our mothers didn't have Teflon, but somehow they managed, and there weren't as many diseases then as we constantly hear about today. Time spent on keeping you healthy is time well spent.

Are Your Plastic Containers Safe?

Now that we have an idea about the foods that are good for us and the foods that aren't, let's look at what we're storing our food in. Many of the plastic bottles (including bottled-water bottles) and containers on the market are not safe; they are made with toxic materials that can have a negative effect on health.

On the bottom of most plastic bottles and containers, you will find a number within a triangle. These numbers indicate the safety of the plastic. Use the guidelines below to see whether your plastic containers are safe. BPA (Bisphenol A) is used to make many plastic bottles and is also used to make epoxy resins. According to Wikipedia, BPAs have been suspected of being hazardous to humans since their invention in the 1930s.

The following plastics are not made from Bisphenol A and are considered safe.

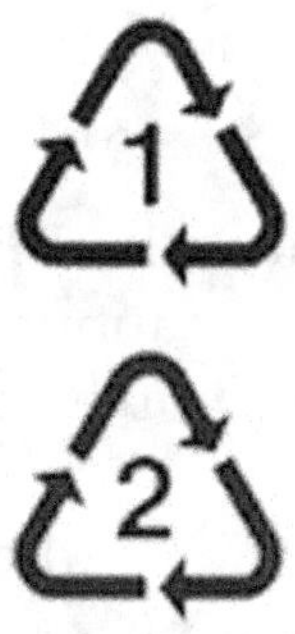

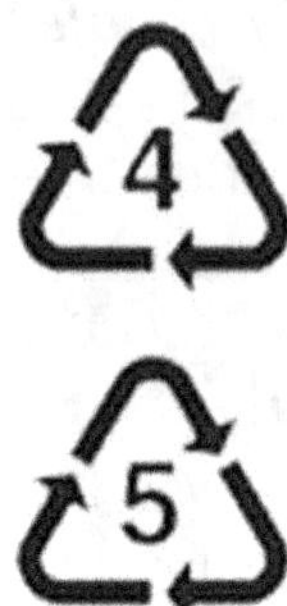

The next numbers, although often found in baby bottles and sippy cups, are unsafe. ***Do not use them***. They are made with Bisphenol A.

Bed Bath and Beyond sells BPA-free 24-piece food storage container sets for about twenty dollars. Always look for reusable water bottles that say "BPA free."

Knowledge is power, and when it comes to your health, ignorance is not bliss. You should know what you are eating and what you are putting your food in.

Chapter 10

Invest in Your Body, Invest in Your Life

I know I've given you a lot of information. But the changes we've looked at do not need to be made overnight. Of course, the sooner you make these changes, the better. Ultimately, you need to make these changes in a way that is going to work for your lifestyle.

When I decided to change my lifestyle, I tackled one challenge at a time. I always enjoyed exercise, so for me that was a perfect place to start. Next I changed my eating habits—in steps. First I gave up hydrogenated oils, then high fructose corn syrup. From there I eliminated as much white flour as I could from my diet and started eating whole grains.

After I made all of my dietary changes, I started looking at the way I prepare foods. The microwave was the first thing to go. It was years before I discovered the convection oven, but I finally did. Then I got rid of my non-stick pans. It was quite some time before Cuisinart came out with the Greenware line. You should have seen how terrible my whole-wheat pancakes looked cooking in my aluminum pans, but that wasn't a priority. My health was more important than how great my pancakes looked.

Fortunately I have come across alternatives since then—and so can you. You can have great-tasting pancakes that look good and don't harm you! You can get rid of your microwave and still save a little bit of time by using a convection oven. I didn't get rid of my microwave until I knew that I was no longer dependent on it. Much to my surprise, it only took a couple of weeks to adjust to life without the microwave. I wasn't even sure I could live without it. Now, I don't miss it at all.

Health is such an amazing gift. Who would ever want to turn down an amazing *free* gift? The natural aging process takes a toll on the body, true, but don't add additional stress to your life by putting off good health and great food. Invest in your body, invest in your life.

Remember, 30 percent of how you age is genetics. The rest is up to you!